Diagnosis:
BRAIN TUMOR

23.5 Hours to a Miracle

✞

RICK JONES

Eden Publishing

© Copyright 2000 by Rick Jones.

All Rights Reserved. No part of this book may be reproduced or transmitted in any form or by any means, electronic or mechanical, including photocopying, recording, or by any information storage or retrieval system, without permission in writing from the author.

Cover Design by Jeff Sharpton, Design Point.

ISBN NO. 1-884898-14-9

Library of Congress Catalog Card No. 99-071229

1. Brain tumor   2. Acoustic Neuroma   3. Changed Life
4. Forgiveness   5. Recovery

To book author for speaking engagements, or to obtain additional copies of this book, address:

Rick Jones, 635 N. Terry Street, Portland, OR 97217
(503) 735-3133 - e-mail: rick23.5@juno.com

This book was published through arrangement with author and distributed by Eden Publishing, P. O. Box 20176, Keizer, OR 97307-0176.

To the three women who helped
make this book possible.

Kay Lee
LeeAnn Jones
Barbara Dan

And my deep graditude to:
Dr. Tanabe, who went the distance.
Dr. Canepe, who took a chance.
Dr. Montgomery, who renewed my mind.

CHAPTER 1.

At first I wouldn't admit I had a problem. Now I can look back and realize that the symptoms were there for at least three years. For a year the symptoms had been bad, yet somehow I managed to ignore them. Like most American men I was taught to be tough. "If you just ignore it and keep working, it will go away."

However, my problems just weren't going away. When I lifted things, I would get a severe headache, a headache so bad that I would fall to my knees. I noticed my vision was becoming progressively worse. When I looked out of the corner of my eyes, my eyeballs would twitch. I was having trouble with my balance. I would stumble at night, if I didn't have anything to focus on. I was losing strength on my left side. When I held the phone my left arm would twitch, and my wife said I was shaking at night. I finally had to admit that something was wrong and I needed to quit being macho and do something about it.

At the time I was working for a company where I finally felt at home, and I was working for a person I respected. I was hoping for some peace in my life. I had grown up in the midst of turmoil. While I was growing up, my father's addiction to alcohol kept him away most of the time. When I was ten, my parents divorced and I was robbed of my father completely. Until age sixteen I only saw him one day out of every six months. At sixteen I started to drink on a regular basis. I dropped out of high school and went to the Oregon coast to work with my dad as a commercial fisherman.

For the next three years I worked hard and drank even harder. When I wasn't fishing, I worked as a logger or in the lumber mills. Eventually my drinking took over my life. I attempted to solve my problems by moving back to Portland where I met my wife. After a brief courtship we were married in October of 1988. I had gone to church as a boy, and I believed in God. I had accepted Jesus as my savior when I was nineteen, but I struggled with my relationship with God and with my wife. My marriage was filled with a great deal of stress which I tried to avoid with drinking binges.

I began working long hours for a steel company, but I was unhappy about the way they treated their workers. Finally, in 1994 I found a steel company where I was happy. I was working there when I started having physical problems. My wife had a two- year-old-son when we got married, and we had two more children in the next few years. We bought a house and tried to have a good life. I was hoping, now that I had a good job, that everything would fall into place. On my twenty-sixth birthday I decided to quit drinking once and for all, and I haven't gotten drunk since.

I was putting a lot of energy into my career and my family. My wife and kids were important; I needed to pay attention to them, and also try to move forward at work. I was trying to find a balance between these two forces so I could find peace. At the same time, I had physical problems, but no time or energy to deal with them. Stubbornly, I continued to ignore my symptoms or wish them away. I decided that the problem was my back. I had not seen a doctor. Someone suggested that I go see a chiropractor. When I did, the chiropractor told me that my back was out of alignment.

Being young and inexperienced, I let him adjust me and he sent me on my way. My problems didn't go away. So I returned. He adjusted my back again and told me I was probably going to be sore for awhile. He said my back had been out so long it would take some time for it to fall back into place.

Looking back, I realize I should have asked more questions. I should have asked, "Why don't we take x-rays?" Instead, I felt frustrated and foolish for going to the chiropractor. I decided I needed to quit whining. Besides, the chiropractor was expensive so I didn't go back.

One Saturday I was working on top of an eight foot high steel rack. When I went to lift a bar of steel, a headache came on so strong and so quickly that I almost fell off the rack. I dropped the bar of steel, fell to my knees, and hung on desperately to the rack until everything came back in focus. I climbed down and told my coworker, Dean, that I needed to go see a chiropractor.

I was still hoping they could cure me. I found one that was open on a Saturday that would take my insurance, so I went. He listened to what I had to say, put some vibrating devices on my back for awhile, adjusted me and sent me on my way with no medications and no follow-up plan. The treatment didn't help so I decided I would just have to live with the pain until I could get a desk job.

One day as I was driving home from work, the pain in my neck was so intense I thought I would pass out. My sinuses were clogged, my vision was really bad, and my head ached so much I couldn't turn my neck. I was almost home when I saw a chiropractor's office. I whipped into the parking lot. I could hardly walk from the truck to the door. This clinic wasn't covered by my insurance, but the chiropractor was so sure he could help me that I paid for the visits out of my own pocket.

I told him what kind of shape I was in, and he took me back to an examination room. He was very friendly and talked a lot. He gave me a whole spiel about diet, stretching and exercise. He said that my back had been out of adjustment for a long time and he couldn't fix it in one visit. I would need to come see him for several sessions.

He adjusted me and set me up with four appointments, once a week in advance. I kept all the appointments. During one visit I asked him, "What about x-rays? None of the chiropractors have taken x-rays of me."

He told me if he couldn't fix the problem, then he would take an x-ray. I took the initiative and set up an appointment with a radiology clinic that was covered by my insurance. I called the chiropractor and he told me, "Let's not do the x-ray yet. Come in for another session."

I said okay and went in for one more session, but I still wasn't feeling that good. I had spent about two hundred dollars, and I still owed him money. I went home and my wife asked me how I felt. I think I told her I felt better because I didn't want her to get mad at me and start saying, "Geez, you just spent two hundred dollars on this chiropractor and it isn't doing you any good." So I quit going to him, too, for about three weeks.

Things at home were hectic. My wife was stressed out from running her day care business and didn't want to believe there was anything wrong. I continued to try and hold things together.

As I look back to that time in my life, I can remember a lot of inward struggles. I guess they were more like battles. Not only was I dealing with physical problems that I didn't know the cause of, but I was dealing with questions that a lot of us are trying to answer. Questions like, "Who am I?" "What do I really believe?" "What's important to me, and how am I going to live my life?" It was a time when some things were coming together and some things were falling apart. It became clear to me that I needed to do a lot of thinking and find some answers that would work for my life.

CHAPTER 2

Finally, the symptoms could no longer be ignored. I was making deliveries; driving a steel truck at that time was a big part of my job. I remember thinking, *I am liable for all this steel, and if I get one of my massive headaches while I am behind the wheel, and pass out, I could kill somebody. There are women and kids out there I could hurt, so I need to find out what the problem is.* I knew now that something was desperately wrong and that I wasn't just complaining.

I made an appointment with my wife's doctor. I couldn't get in to see anyone else. She happened to be on duty at the evening clinic that night. I told her all the problems I was having and all the chiropractic adjustments I had had. I said, "You know, I have been to chiropractors, and once I went to the emergency room with facial paralysis and they told me it was anxiety. There is something wrong and I don't want to go away from here feeling foolish that I ever came to see a doctor in the first place."

She tested me, and right away I sensed that she knew

something was wrong. She went through a series of tests, and as she gave each test the expression on her face went from polite professional concern to a puzzled concern. She told me to get dressed and she said that I definitely had nystagmus, which is a rapid involuntary eye movement, my balance was off, I had resting tremors, and it looked to her like the left side of my face was starting to droop. She told me that she was just a general practitioner, she didn't know what was wrong but she wanted me to see Dr. Rosenbaum, a neurologist.

The next day I called Dr. Rosenbaum's office for an appointment and they couldn't get me in for two weeks. I remember feeling frustrated. I went back to work and told the boss I had an appointment in two weeks with a neurologist. I was thinking, *Boy, they will probably find a back problem or nerve damage.*

Back at work, the headaches were constant now. Sometimes when I was in a hurry I would stop the truck, put the brakes on and jump down real quick to go untie my load, and the headaches would start. Or I would just laugh and the headaches would start. So I called Dr. Rosenbaum's office and told them about the headaches to see if I could get an earlier appointment, but they just didn't have any openings. I was frustrated about this, but because I was a young man, looked upon as being healthy and strong, I felt like I was whining. What if I made a big stink and got in earlier and they didn't find anything wrong? I would be embarrassed. So I said okay and decided I would just tough it out.

Finally the day for the neurologist's visit arrived. I usually loaded the truck that day so I could leave early in the morning to drive to Eugene about 100 miles south of Portland, Oregon, where I live. I told my boss I needed to go see a neurologist and I really didn't think that I should be driving anymore. He agreed to take me off driving until after I had seen the neurologist.

My appointment was in the afternoon, and Dr. Robert Rosenbaum examined me. He did a series of tests. He touched my eye with a Kleenex and my left eye would not blink. He did sensation tests on my face and on my legs and arms. Then he excused himself for a minute and walked out of the room.

He came back shortly with a younger man. He explained that this was a neurological intern who was working with him. He told the intern that I was a 27- year- old white male in relatively healthy condition. He explained that I had nystagmus of the eye, left side weakness and loss of sensation in the left eye. He let the intern examine me and then they left the room.

When Dr. Rosenbaum came back in he said, "Well, there are three things we can do. One, I can send you for an MRI. Two, I can send you for a CTI or three, I can just send you home and wait and see if these problems resolve themselves.

Sometimes we don't find anything wrong. What I want to do is send you in for an MRI but it is your choice. I want to send you in right away. You're a young man and sometimes young people's neurological problems go away, but I want you to come in tomorrow. I can't get you in tonight."

I said, "Okay, that's fine." I went home, thinking, *Why doesn't he do the CTI because the CTI is for the neck and the spinal cord. The MRI is for the brain.* Of course, he was the neurologist and I wasn't about to argue with him.

When I told my wife about the tests, she didn't seem particularly concerned. I told her I thought I had some neck problems from when a pipe fell on my head back in 1990. I had sustained some neck damage and had gone to physical therapy for it.

The next day I went to work like any other day. I told my supervisor I needed to leave for an MRI. I remember it was a very busy day and I could tell that he was concerned. We had discussed on several occasions about going to the doctor and being sent home because there was nothing wrong. My supervisor had a grand mal seizure once, and the doctors never did find out what was wrong with him. We both did not have a lot of faith in the medical field.

I called Dr. Rosenbaum's office around nine o'clock in the morning and the receptionist told me an MRI was scheduled for ten thirty. I told my supervisor that I needed to go for an

MRI at ten thirty and I probably would be back by noon. I could see relief on his face that I wouldn't be gone all day.

I finished up a few things and drove down to the hospital where I filled out the usual paperwork. The staff asked me if I had any metal in my body, and I told them I had a metal splinter in my eye about six months before this. So they took me down the hall for an eye x-ray.

I waited in the lobby until a technician came and took me to the MRI scanning room. He gave me a gown and a robe. He explained their procedures. He said I would be put in the tube; later I would have dye injected into my veins and a further series of x-rays would be done.

They put me in the tube and there was a lot of clunk, clunk, clunk, clunk noise. I remember thinking it had taken about as long as they said it would. I wondered when were they going to take me out and put the dye in my veins. Then I heard the machine go on again, taking more pictures. I was thinking, *This is kinda curious.* When they were finally finished, the technician walked over to me and looked at me with a sober look on his face. He was very professional, but I could sense that something unusual was happening. He said, "I'm going to put the dye in your arm now."

He put the dye in my arm and went back out. I was in the MRI tube quite awhile. They took a series of pictures; then finally they pulled me out and told me I could get dressed.

The technician said, "I want you to wait in the lobby." I asked him if I was free to go, and he said, "No, I have to call your doctor and talk to him before I let you go." That struck me as curious so I walked out to the lobby and telephoned my wife.

I told her I was done with the MRI scans and that they wanted me to wait until they contacted my doctor. I was a bit puzzled. She also thought it was strange that it took two weeks to get in to see Dr. Rosenbaum, yet all of a sudden they wanted me to wait until the technician could talk to him. Maybe they had found something. I agreed with her, but I had no idea what they could have found.

I got off the phone with my wife and called my boss. I told him that I couldn't leave the hospital yet. It could take a while, because they had to talk to my doctor. I promised to call him as soon as I could come back to work and I hung up the phone.

Finally the technician came out and told me that Dr. Rosenbaum wanted to see me in his office at one o'clock. At that point, I wouldn't say that I started to get alarmed, but I started getting serious. I knew that it was out of the ordinary. I knew that for Dr. Rosenbaum to see me on such short notice, they must have found something.

I thought they had found nerve damage and wanted to tell me I couldn't go back to work. So I went and ate lunch.

CHAPTER 3

I arrived at Dr. Rosenbaum's office at about quarter to one. His office is in the Providence Portland Medical Center building. I sat there nervous and a little anxious until Dr. Rosenbaum came out and took me back to his office. He told me to sit down, he sat on the edge of the desk and confirmed my suspicions: "We found something."

From the look on his face I could tell that it wasn't good. Still, I told myself, *It can't be that bad because he only said that 'we found something.'*

He took me over to the MRI scans and began to show me the x-rays as he explained in medical terminology. It didn't seem that serious to me. He showed me the x-rays from this angle and from that angle. He showed me how far the spot went down and how deep it was. Then he showed me an x-ray that was a shot from the back of the brain. That's when I really saw it. He said, "It's a tumor."

When he said that, it really shocked me.

I looked at him and asked, "How bad is it?" He showed

me the brain stem with the tumor right against the brain stem. It was actually pushing the brain stem over about a half-inch, so that the brain stem was curved.

He said, "It's a rather large tumor. But it's not that, it's the location. It's in the crevice of your brain on the brain stem. I'm not a surgeon, but it looks like a benign tumor. It's probably not cancerous. It looks like a uniform tumor. It should just come right out of there. Again, I am not a brain surgeon. You need to go see one immediately. As a matter of fact, I am going to call Dr. Schmidt right now. He's upstairs, he's a very good surgeon and I'll send you right up. The surgeon has to make the final decision, but in my opinion it has to come out."

He explained that surgery was the only option, because there are two ventricles in the brain that produce brain fluid and one of these was almost shut off because of the tumor. Doctors can't determine exactly how fast tumors grow, but it seemed to him that if the tumor grew even a half of a centimeter larger it would shut that ventricle off completely, causing a buildup of fluid in my brain and I would die. This could happen in maybe three to six months.

At that point it hit me. I said, "My God, this is serious!" Dr. Rosenbaum called the surgeon and while I sat there in a daze, he talked to Dr. Schmidt in medical terms. He suggested I call some family to meet me in Dr. Schmidt's office.

I remember walking out into the hallway in a state of shock. I took the elevator up one floor and gave my name to Dr. Schmidt's secretary. She told me to have a seat and I asked her if I could use the phone to call my wife. When Melanie picked up the phone I told her she needed to get there right away. When she asked me why, I told her, "I have a brain tumor," then I started crying.

"God, no, you're kidding me," she responded. I told her I wasn't kidding and she needed to come right away because I was waiting to see the brain surgeon in his office. She said, "Okay, I'll get there as soon as I can."

Next, I called work. When Linda, the secretary answered, I told her, "I don't think I will be coming in tomorrow. In fact, I don't think I'll be coming in anymore at all."

She asked me what was wrong and I explained that they found a brain tumor and I was at the brain surgeon's office. I began crying again and I was glad that no one else was in the waiting room.

The secretary asked me something else, but I couldn't answer. I had my head down on my hands, and I broke down and wept. I couldn't believe it. I was only twenty-seven years old. Things like this just don't happen to me. I had three children.

In the back of my mind I kept thinking, it can't be that serious. My wife came in with a panicked look on her face.

She sat down and started asking me about the tumor and I just said it was on the brain stem and I had to see the surgeon, but other than that I didn't know a lot.

I got a phone call from my mother. My wife had called her before she came. The secretary handed me the phone, and my mom asked me if I was okay. Then she told me, "We're not going to ask each other that anymore. Of course, you're not okay." I explained to her that I was at the surgeon's office and I asked her to come.

When it was time to see the surgeon, he had me get into a gown and performed a very lengthy examination. He checked my coordination, the movement of my hands and eyes. The doctor was in his mid-fifties, serious, with a tall slender build. After I dressed, we went into his office. My wife and I sat looking at each other with very scared looks on our faces.

By that time my mother and two brothers had arrived. We all sat there in silence as the surgeon examined my x-rays for about fifteen minutes. He examined them closely while making notes. He was a very calm, precise man.

Finally, he sat on the edge of the desk. I can't remember his exact words but he told us that I had a large tumor in a difficult place. It was pressing against the brain stem, probably benign, but he wouldn't know until he biopsied it.

He warned us of the risks connected with this surgery. They ranged from facial paralysis to being comatose, or even death. I had no other options. The tumor had to come out. It was too large for chemotherapy or radiation.

He told us to go home but not to delay in deciding. He also suggested I write my last will and testament and take care of anything else that needed to be set in order. He told us he would contact us the following week.

My mother and my brothers were very worried. As we walked out together, I slung my arm around one of my brothers. My mom asked what I wanted to do and I told her I didn't know. I suggested we go out for pizza, it was all I could think of. I think we stopped in the hallway. My wife was crying. I don't think it had hit all of us yet. I rode with my wife. My brother drove my truck home.

CHAPTER 4

I immediately started calling people. I called my dad and left a message on his machine. I called my uncle Bill. All he could say was, "I am sorry to hear that." He's always been very positive man. He told me he would see me before the operation and that everything would be okay. At that platitude we both laughed.

My brother Thom, his wife and baby, my mom and my brother Steve, along with my wife and kids, went out to pizza and surprisingly we just talked. No one knew what to say. There was a real soberness in the air. I almost felt like it was the Last Supper, as if I had been given my death sentence. I definitely never thought anything like this would ever happen to me. About eight o'clock we went home. I just wanted to be with my wife and my kids.

The phone was ringing when we walked in the door. It was my father. I asked how he was doing and he told me he was sick because he had been talking about me with Uncle Bill. I explained to him about my tumor and that it was on the brain stem in a very bad place. He said he would come as soon as possible.

Growing up, I had felt a lot of bitterness and hatred towards my father because I felt he had abandoned me. All that changed. None of it mattered anymore. All that mattered was that he was my dad, I loved him and all I could think was, *Gee, I hope I get to see him again.* I felt like it was time to put things behind me and to stop carrying a grudge.

After my wife and I put the kids to bed, we went to bed. My wife just laid there and cried. We held each other tight. She kept saying, "I can't believe this is happening. It seems like a bad dream." I felt very close to her

I thought how having a wife was a serious commitment and the wedding vows came to my mind, "through sickness and health till death do us part." I had promised to love and cherish her, yet I had ambitions. Like a lot of men, I faltered in the growth and maturity it takes to sacrifice and give yourself to love someone.

The next day Melanie's mother called, and offered to pay for us to go to the coast for the weekend. We went, but it was hard to enjoy myself, because my headache was so terrible and because I couldn't shut out what was going on. It was a very stressful weekend, but we tried to enjoy it the best that we could.

When we drove back into town on Monday, the first thing we did was call the doctor. I was getting quite nervous and upset, because he hadn't called and nearly a week had passed.

My wife talked to the doctor and listening to my wife's conversation, I realized that the doctor wasn't going to do the operation. He told my wife that after examining the x-rays and doing more research, he had decided it would be too difficult for him. He said it would take him two surgeries to get it all out. He wanted to refer us to another doctor. The fear of dying became real to me.

From the time we got home from the coast the phone began to ring off the hook. Friends were calling, trying to encourage me. Most of them told me that things were going to be just fine, that I would have the operation and feel great.

The next Saturday I decided to rent all six Star Trek movies. Because I am a big Star Trek fan, I watched all six of them, in hopes of getting my mind off the brain tumor. Having a whole Saturday to myself and watching them didn't bring the satisfaction I hoped for.

At night it would be one or two in the morning before we could fall asleep. My wife and I would just lie there and think and sometimes she would cry. We were both scared and we held each other a lot. In my heart, whether it was just me, or God was speaking to me, I felt like it was not going to be just fine. I felt I was going to live, but that I would never be the same.

It wasn't going to be just a simple operation.

CHAPTER 5

Dr. Schmidt referred us to Dr. Tanabe. The tumor was next to a very delicate area of the brain stem. Dr. Tanabe was reputed to be one of the best brain surgeons around. We got an appointment in a just a few days.

Dr. Tanabe took his time examining me. I immediately took a liking to him. He made me feel at ease. He went over my MRI scans with my wife and me. He told us my tumor was an acoustic neuroma. He said that it was rare for a man my age to have a tumor that large, and that they only occur in about five people out of every million. He estimated the tumor had been growing there for about seven years.

Dr. Tanabe went on to say that I would definitely lose the hearing in my left ear and that I would have left-sided facial paralysis. These were a given. I could also have paralysis in my left arm and my left leg, possibly even coma or death. I would also have problems with the vision in my left eye.

Using a sculpture of the brain, Dr. Tanabe explained where he would go in and what he would do. He would have to remove a portion of the left side cerebellum to get to the tumor. They would not be able to put back all of the bone, because the point of entry was so low in the skull. I would have a hole in my head the rest of my life, but it would be covered by neck muscles.

My wife asked him if we could get a second opinion. He told us we were more than welcome to get one, but he didn't know where to refer us, because he was the only doctor around who was both qualified to operate on me and willing to do it. His exact words to me were, "I may be crazy, but I like a challenge."

In a way this comforted me, because I knew he was being honest. On the other hand, it scared me to have to face how serious this was. The knowledge that I was facing a very tough battle began to be a strong reality for me.

Another brain surgeon, Dr. Rohrer, would be assisting Dr. Tanabe. He introduced him and I really liked him, too. The surgery was scheduled to take place in two weeks. The tumor had been there for a long time, and I was told that a delay of a month or two would be too long, but a couple of weeks wouldn't make a difference. He said to call if my symptoms worsened.

One morning my headache became very severe. I was

staggering around, and my wife had to help me down the stairs. I called the doctor, and he prescribed a steroid to bring down the swelling in the brain. All of my symptoms seemed to be getting worse and my energy level was low.

Later that week the surgeon's office called and told me my surgery date was May 3rd. I was to report in at five a.m. Surgery would begin at eight a.m. Having the date set was a confirmation that this was real.

The next two weeks I spent time with my wife and my kids. I went out to the job site and talked to Mike, my boss. He was very upset. At one point I even saw tears come to his eyes. Mike said he would do everything in his power financially to help. He said for right now I was on medical leave and that I would get my full pay, vacation pay and bonuses as long as possible. This took a big load off my mind.

I went to some prayer meetings and asked people to pray for me. At one prayer meeting they were praying about the gang problems in North Portland. I remember feeling that having surgery is a big deal to me, but a lot more important things were going on that were more needy than me. After all, I had medical insurance and a family that loved me. I had the best brain surgeon in Portland working on me. I had reason to be upset, but I didn't have enough reason to feel sorry for myself.

People came and talked to me, and I told them, "If I am

disabled after this surgery I can live with it. It is amazing what you can live with when death is the alternative."

Death was a very real possibility to me. Looking at my children's faces I would think, *I may never see them again. They may grow up without me. They may grow up without a daddy.* I knew my children wouldn't care if I couldn't walk or use my left arm, or if the left side of my face was paralyzed. They would just care if I was there or not, if they could hug me or not.

It was amazing how my view on life changed. I could live with a lot of things. Still, I sensed this was going to be a greater battle than everybody was telling me. People kept assuring me that things would go smoothly, that everything was going to be just fine. I told them, "I don't think so. I think this is going to change my life. I think this is going to be a great battle for me." I struggled to try and keep things in perspective.

CHAPTER 6

When my wife and I would talk at night, I would think, *This is my chance.* I had always relied on my physical attributes to get me by, to build things and take care of business. I hoped this experience would change me so I would finally know what was important in life. I wanted to be able to stand on my principles and see the hand of God work in my life. I thought I was going to be able to live life to the fullest, understand what was important to me, and not have a problem with my temper anymore. I would be the most wonderful father and husband. It sounds kind of foolish, but I was hoping that somehow this experience would fix all of my problems.

I watched TV talk shows and read books about people who went through traumas and how it changed them. I hoped it would fix my relationship with my wife. We sometimes loved each other, sometimes hated each other. We experienced hope and despair, but all in all our marriage was very stressful and needy. Those two weeks before the surgery we were very close. All our fighting and problems seemed to disappear, and I enjoyed it.

The clock ticked away as the day drew nearer. I threw a birthday party for my wife and my younger brother Steve. I wanted to get my wife a gift that would be meaningful. I went to a gem shop and bought a raw amethyst. I wrote on the card, "You are my rock." I gave it to her and told her that no matter what happened after my surgery I wanted the amethyst to be cut and set into a ring. I thought it would be special.

At the birthday party I saw people I hadn't seen in quite awhile. Two brothers, Jeff and James Sutherland, came. Their older brother, Gordon, had died of a brain tumor when he was eighteen. I had seen him after his brain surgery. The surgery was successful, but the cancer had already spread. I had known Gordon and his brothers when we were kids, then lost track of them. I started up a relationship again when he had cancer. Gordon was a good person, got straight A's in school, was a track star, and had a strong commitment to God for his age. He was a moral person. I, on the other hand, was not a shining example.

Once, I stayed with Gordon for a month. We went to Bible camp together and that is when I got saved. After a month with Gordon, I went back home, to my old neighborhood, to my old friends. For a while I followed my convictions, but I soon fell back into my old ways. I began getting into trouble. I was an angry person and my life ran in cycles. I went through the stage, I don't care; the hell with the world I can do what I want. I drank, and got in fights. I would then hit a wall, feel remorseful, and look for a way out.

Seeing Jeff and James brought back these memories. Right to the end Gordon's faith was steady. He knew God was going to heal him. There was no doubt in his mind, yet he died. This hurt me deeply, and I got mad at God. I asked God why this person who had so much to offer and was doing well had to suffer and die? It hurt.

I got so tired at the party that as the night wore on I began to see double. Emotionally I was drained. We sent people home and went to bed, only to toss and turn until two a.m., trying to fall asleep so we could get up at seven. My entire working life I had dreamed of having more time to spend at home. I wanted to be there when my kids came home from school. Now my chance had finally come, and I couldn't even enjoy it.

I did have a few brief moments of enjoyment being home; then reality would come crashing down on me. My relationship with my wife was good at that point, better than it ever had been. In the past I had an anger problem, so that even though I never hit my wife, I would yell a lot. We lived in constant stress, trying to collect possessions and do fun activities too fast without building the foundations of marriage and family. This kept us too busy to focus on ourselves.

The whole week before surgery I walked around in a daze. The steroids made me hungry so I ate a lot. I enjoyed visiting with people I didn't see that often. My uncle came by and took me out to breakfast, and we talked like we never had before. We talked about the distance between us and the fact that our family didn't see each other unless something bad happened, or there was a death in the family.

I decided that even if I lost the use of a leg or an arm or both, I would learn to live with that and enjoy my family. I was getting a whole new view of things.

I went to see my grandparents and their response was from the old school: Keep a stiff upper lip. Everything would be okay.

I took lots of vitamins to build my system up.

I was scared, but I just knew I was going to live through this surgery.

I wasn't reading my Bible or praying every day, but I felt close to God. I realized God really did love me unconditionally. Basically it came down to this: Do I believe that Jesus died for my sins and forgave me? Do I accept His forgiveness, or do I not believe? All that mattered was knowing that if I did die, I would be in heaven. I was comforted, too, because if I did die, I would be under the anesthesia and I wouldn't have to feel panic at the thought of dying.

I knew I was preparing for battle. I was like a warrior taking stock of his weaponry. It was physical, it was mental, it was spiritual, a battle within. It was a tough battle to wage. When you face off with an opponent, your objective is to win. When you are facing off with yourself, it is difficult, because you can't just shut off your thoughts. I battled constantly with feelings of terror. I felt sorry for myself, I felt sorry for my wife, I felt sorry for my kids.

I went down and ate lunch at school with Bryon, my oldest. He really enjoyed having me there. He got wound up and told his friends, "Look, my dad is here. My dad has a brain tumor. He has to go to the hospital and get his head cut open." It was blunt but refreshingly honest.

May 2nd came, the day before surgery, my wife and I had an appointment with Dr. Tanabe. He sat down with us. "This is a big surgery," he said, "and I want you here very early in the morning at five a.m. I don't need to go over the risks with you. I have already explained them."

I asked a few questions, such as what it would be like afterwards. He told me he really wasn't sure. He expected the surgery to be eight to twelve hours. Then I would be in ICU and in a lot of pain for a couple days. After that, I would move to acute care for about a week. Then I could go home.

Dr. Tanabe was a big source of encouragement to me. He didn't make a big deal of things, but I could tell that this surgery had him worried. I could see it even though he was doing all he could to keep a professional posture.

My wife and I left the appointment with a real sense of soberness. We held each other's hand. There wasn't much to say. We drove to my mother's where my grandma and grandpa were staying. My mother fixed us dinner. My dad and step-mom were at my house, taking care of my kids. My mom and grandma were very positive in front of me, but I would catch them crying. It was tough. I helped my grandpa fix the RV.

We went home, talked to my dad for awhile and put the kids to bed. I went to lay down and amazingly enough, I fell right to sleep. I had to be up at four in the morning, and this was the first time I had slept soundly. I was dead asleep when my wife woke me up at four. She went to get her sister, who was going to watch the kids. When she returned I was still asleep and she had to wake me again. We agreed not to wake the kids.

CHAPTER 7

I got up and took a quick shower. By five a.m. I was ready to go. I started to panic, because my wife was walking around doing meaningless little jobs I kept saying, "Come on, Honey. We've got to go."

It took us until five-twenty to get out the door. I was so anxious about not being late. I look back now and realize how silly that was. It was like worrying about being late to your own funeral.

We got to the hospital and my mom was there. I checked in and went up to the 7th floor. It was all very calm. I was just sitting there, and my dad and step-mom came in and we talked small talk. No one knew what to say.

The nurses came in and out and prepped me. At seven thirty they came with a gurney, and told me it was time to go. I had this burning feeling in my chest, as if someone had started a fire. It was slowly growing.

They put me on the gurney and this very friendly attendant named Bob began talking to me as they wheeled me down the hallway. My mother and my dad followed close behind, and my wife was there beside me.

At the door to the pre-op room, only one person could go in with me. I said good-bye to my dad, and he hugged me and told me that he loved me.

I said good-bye to my step-mom and then my mother. I remember looking at them as long as I could. I was thinking, *I may never see them again.* I wondered if they realized they might never see their boy again. I have children, and I wouldn't want to watch one of my kids get wheeled away.

In pre-op they put me in a very small room. My wife sat with me, holding my hand. I was real nervous. Dr. Evans, the anesthesiologist, came in. I took a liking to him right away and felt he was someone good, who actually cared and wasn't doing his job just for the money. He was very efficient and took time to explain the risks to me, while he put an arterial IV in. He numbed my arm, but it hurt like you wouldn't believe, because it was deep. Then he gave me something to calm me down.

The nurses came and took my blood pressure. Then a lady chaplain came and asked if I wanted her to pray for me. I don't remember what she prayed, but it made me feel better. Then it was time to go. I faced another set of doors and my wife kissed me and told me things would be okay. I knew they wouldn't. I looked at my wife and thought that I didn't deserve her, and I didn't know what I would do without her. I squeezed her hand and told her I loved her and then, all of a sudden, there I was among strangers.

We went through two sets of doors and down a long hallway and it was very cold. They wheeled me into the operating room and it was even colder. I started shivering, partly because I was cold and partly because I was afraid.

All of a sudden that burning coal in my chest exploded. I saw Dr. Tanabe standing in the middle of the room with a lot of other people. It was a big room. In the middle of the room stood a stainless steel table. Beside it were what looked like two big Snap-On tool boxes. Air hoses were hanging from the ceiling and a giant light hovered over the table. It looked more like an automotive shop than an operating room.

They stopped the gurney and said it was time to transfer me. Obediently, I stood up and walked across the floor. Dr. Tanabe was standing there with his arms behind his back. Everyone else was rushing around, while Dr. Tanabe just stood there like a general overseeing the battlefield. He was watching everyone, yet he paused and said hello to me. He introduced me to the scrub nurse and I said, "Hi."

Dr. Rohrer was on the telephone. I thought that was interesting. Dr. Tanabe introduced me to the neurosurgery team, and I looked at them. I felt like I did when I was a child and had my tonsils out. When it was time to go to surgery I had tried to climb out a window. I didn't see a window to climb out this time. He told me very solemnly, "It's time to get on the table now."

As I laid back on the table, I began shivering uncontrollably. I felt as if someone had turned on a switch and turned me into a jack hammer. Dr. Evans started covering me with heated blankets and then put something in my IV that spread the most incredible warmth over me.

Dr. Tanabe walked over, patted me on the shoulder, and just looked at me. He didn't say anything. He just looked at me and nodded his head. He could see that I was terrified. I had thought I would feel close to God and prayerful, but my mind went blank and fear just took over. I could see the bright lights and the surgery team looking at me. Then Dr. Evans put me out. It was like being dropped down a black hole where the light gets smaller and smaller and then everything is just black.

CHAPTER 8

The next thing I remember was waking up. I couldn't see anything except a blur of bright lights, but I could tell I was still in the operating room. I could feel them working on my head. I heard a loud humming that sounded like a giant laser gun. I remember thinking, *My God, they're not done yet! I'm waking up!* I was terrified that any moment I was going to start feeling them operating on me. Then I went back out.

I woke up again. The room was dark, but I knew I was somewhere in the hospital. I bit down and could feel something in my mouth. At the time all I could think was, *It hasn't been long enough. They stopped because they had problems and couldn't operate anymore and I am going to die.* I felt panic and hopelessness. The feeling was total terror. The room was dark, and I was very disoriented. I felt like there was a group of people laughing at me, and I wondered why these people were laughing. I thought they were trying to kill me, and I began to struggle. I remember my arms were bound and I fought to get something out of my mouth. Again, I went out.

When I came to again I was very sick. I threw up and then lots of nurses clustered around me holding my arms and legs. One of the nurses stuck something down my throat and began suctioning me. I remember her telling me, "Cough, Rick, cough." I coughed and she told me, "Good job, Rick, good job."

This must be what it feels like to drown, I thought. I tried to take in air. I couldn't because my lungs had fluid in them. I felt like I was dying, and no one would do anything.

I could faintly hear my wife talking. She was telling me I had been in surgery for almost twenty four hours, but I was going to be okay. They had got it all out.

When she told me I had been in surgery for almost twenty four hours, it began to dawn on me that I was messed up pretty bad. I tried to move my arms and legs. They wouldn't move. I had double vision and couldn't see. I tried to focus and got extremely exhausted.

There was a loud noise in my head. It was if someone had laid me next to a train track when a train was going by. Sometimes the noise was unbearable. I kept wondering, *Why did they put me so close to the freeway? Why don't they do something about the noise?* When I tried to talk, all that would come out was gurgling. I could hear, but barely, because the noise in my head was so loud. Even my thoughts bounced back and forth between reality and illusion.

Various relatives began to come in. I remember my grandfather grabbing my foot. Grandfather Soderlund was a big man who had lived with pain all of his life due to a back injury that had disabled him. He represented a symbol of strength to me. He grabbed my foot and talked to me softly like I had never heard him talk before. He told me it would be okay I wish he realized how much comfort that brought me. My other grandpa came in, another man I looked up to for strength. It meant a lot to me. My grandma, my father, and my mother came.

Melanie brought the kids in. My daughter looked at me with a blank expression on her face. I could tell she was upset and didn't know what to do. The person lying there with his eyes rolling around, not able to move or respond, and barely able to squeeze her hand didn't look like her Daddy anymore.

I whispered to her, "Girl, how I love you." My feelings were strong but the simplest expressions for me were exhausting. Just to look at someone for a few minutes and gurgle out a few words made me feel as if I had just run a marathon.

The pain. The pain was like something I have never experienced in my life. I have broken my hands; I have fallen out of trees but I was not prepared for this kind of pain. I would panic thinking I was having a heart attack. The nurses would come in, or my wife would be there, and they would tell me I was fine. I tried to believe them, but my mind was telling me the heart attack was real.

CHAPTER 9

Sometimes I felt like my body was being filled up with air. The pressure from within was incredible. I didn't understand. Sometimes I would just scream inside my head. I began having dreams, and I had a hard time telling if they were real or not.

The dream that scared me the most was where I was in hell among many demons. One demon I identified as Satan. All the other demons hated him, but they obeyed him out of fear. I remember thinking, *God, I wish I could kill him.*

One of the demons challenged him; the challenger was a big, mean looking demon. It was like they were Claymation, yet they were made out of stone. I saw the challenger and I thought, *Surely, this one is going to kill Satan.* I was sitting there cheering him on, as he challenged Satan. I thought, *Yeah, now you're in for it. This one's going to kill you.* The demon and Satan engaged in combat. Swiftly and abruptly, Satan picked up a sword and ran it through his heart, and the demon was dead.

I realized it wasn't the end, because after Satan had killed the demon, they all turned and looked at me, and I was alone. He was coming after me next, because I had sided with the challenger. Then I woke up, terrified, because I thought it was real. I thought, *Why doesn't anyone believe me?*

I dreamed that I was back in surgery Dr. Tanabe was operating on my younger brother, Steve, instead of me. My brother had agreed to take my place, but he died, and I was screaming, "No, don't take my brother." I woke up asking for him.

I don't know if it was from the morphine or the damage to my brain, but I constantly had the feeling I had been shot into orbit, as if someone had strapped a rocket to my bed and shot me into space. I hung onto the bed with all the strength I had. All I could move were my hands. I also felt like someone had dropped me off a building, and I was falling in reverse. Sometimes I felt as if my bed was standing up on end and I was about to fall out. I felt like I was floating up to the ceiling, and I would tell my wife and my mother to hold me down. They would push on my chest as hard as they could, but it still didn't help.

My doctor explained that I was receiving mixed signals, similar to getting wires crossed. The brain stem controls the whole body. It was swollen and all the nerves had pressure on them. It was amazing. I took it for granted that I could control my mind and distinguish between reality and fantasy. At that point I was stripped of even the ability to rationalize, or to reason. It was terrifying.

The only reassurance I received was when I would call out to God and ask Him to take control. All I had left was my spirit. One time I cried out to God with my spirit for help. I went into a place that was like outer space. I saw a great battle going on between Jesus and the devil. Jesus came to me and told me he was fighting for my soul. I realized that even though I hadn't given myself to God completely, He still hadn't given up on me.

When the pain and confusion became unbearable, I got angry with Dr. Tanabe. I felt that he should have let me die. The next day I refused any more morphine. I thought it was making me sick. Dr. Rohrer had tears in his eyes as he searched for a pain medicine I would accept. He had asked me where my pain level was and I had told him ten, but I was afraid to try anything. Finally we settled on Darvacet. It helped enough to bring my pain down to about a seven and I was able to tolerate it.

I woke up one night and fear came down on me like someone had dropped an anvil on my chest. I thought, *I could be like this the rest of my life.* I remembered Dr. Tanabe had told me before surgery that I could be comatose or paralyzed.

I called for the nurse, and I was crying. She asked what

was wrong, and I told her, "I don't want to be paralyzed for the rest of my life. This is no way to live."

This nurse was so sweet. She told me I wouldn't be paralyzed for the rest of my life. She sat down next to me and held my hand and flipped on the radio to a country station. It just so happened they were playing a song by Randy Travis that my wife and I played at our wedding, "I Will Love You Forever and Ever, Amen." She started singing it, and it was the sweetest sound. I tried to sing as much as I could. She asked if I knew this song, and she put her ear close and I was able to say it was my wedding song.

This was the first surge of emotion besides terror that I had since surgery. I also felt sorrow. Where have the years gone for us? Why couldn't I have done more for my wife? If I was to be incapacitated like this, instead of wonderful years ahead, all she would have would be stress, heartache and burden.

Perhaps this was a time for me to reflect on my life and realize that I hadn't grown up. I had lived in a fantasy, thinking things were okay, that nothing bad was ever going to happen and I would just glide through life. I didn't need to take a stand on anything and I didn't need to make a change. I thought life would just go on, and things would fall into place. It wasn't happening that way.

I could see I had choices on how to live, and what to

believe. I couldn't choose to be born or to die, but I could choose how to live.

I was still bouncing back and forth between reality and fantasy. I remember having a dream that I was inside my brain. An old man with a miner's helmet and a pickax was picking at my brain stem. He just kept picking and picking while I yelled at him to stop. But it was as if he didn't hear me. I woke up and I still felt something pounding on the back of my head. I told my wife there were little men picking at my brain stem and she told me, "No, you're okay. It's not real."

Deep down I suppose I knew, but as I have said before, the ability to rationalize and tell fantasy from reality was gone.

I kept dreaming I was in water, like I was back in the womb and that would comfort me. In one of my dreams, nurses would pick me up with a sling and put me in a therapy pool, and that would take the pressure off. I also dreamed they put me in a wheel chair and rolled me down to the therapy ward. They would roll me into the water in my wheelchair, and I would just scream in delight because the pressure was finally off. I would wake up frustrated and wonder why I was in ICU and not in the therapy pool. I didn't realize the water was just a dream. I wanted my suffering to be over.

CHAPTER 10

Dave, the head nurse, would come in and talk to me. He would shave me and tell me I needed to start talking and never shut up. He told me as soon as I showed signs of getting better they would take me up to the acute care ward. My wife told me that acute care beds had trapeze bars hanging over them to pull yourself up with, and the rooms were bigger. This gave me something to look forward to. I felt that as soon as I was free from ICU, I would just be able to get up and walk out.

Dave found out that I used to be a boxer and had taken some Tai Kwan Do. He held up his hand and asked if I could hit it. I would throw my arm out in a feeble attempt, but I was too weak and I couldn't see his hand because of my double-vision.

My wife brought in a nurse named Cathy who was a body-builder in her spare time. She would have Cathy flex her muscles, and say to me, "Look, Honey. Look how big her muscles are."

They were trying to appeal to my macho side. That part of me was gone at this point. I didn't care anymore. All I wanted to do was get out of ICU.

I finally started drinking on my own. I went to sleep one night and dreamed that God told me to drink cranberry juice. I woke up and asked for cranberry juice, and they gave it to me. They told me to drink it slowly, but I just slurped it down. Soothing and healing, it felt like water flowing through my brain.

I decided that I needed ice. The staff brought ice and put it on the back of my neck. It made the pain worse. It was so strange, it seemed that they couldn't do anything to take the pain away. It was just something I had to endure. It came down to the battle within.

Dr. Tanabe or Dr. Rohrer came in every day. They would hold up two fingers and ask me how many I could see and I would always say four. They had to get real close because I could hardly talk.

I had large pressure sores on my right leg and the right side of my chest from lying on the table so long. The medical staff was so concerned about these sores that they called in Dr. Canepa, a plastic surgeon to look at them. As he changed my dressings he told me about a surgery called a cross-face-nerve-graft. He thought I would be a good candidate.

I would be one of the first in Oregon to receive the original version of this surgery. I had lost the left side of my face to paralysis. The surgical team had to sever the seventh and eighth nerves during the operation.

Dr. Canepa looked at my wounds while he discussed doing surgery that would possibly restore movement to the left side of my face.

He explained he had never done this surgery before. If it worked, it could bring back the left side of my face almost completely. Right then, I couldn't make any decisions. My wife questioned him. The doctor told me that if he was going to do the operation, they needed to do it as soon as possible. Otherwise the muscles on the left side would start to atrophy without any nerve input. Atrophying is basically deterioration of the muscle.

The success rate of this surgery was 50/50. Prior to my case, they had tried it on Bell Palsy patients after the damage had been done and the muscles were atrophied. The doctor felt that if they did my surgery right away, by the time the muscles started to atrophy the grafted nerve would start providing input to the muscles and they would start to come back. During the period between surgeries, I would use a face stimulator; a device which sent electrical impulses to the muscles and made them contract.

I had trouble grasping all of this. My wife was

investigating different surgeries and would talk to me about them. It was a struggle to understand all of this. I still couldn't make any decisions.

As the days went by in ICU, my wife kept trying to tell me what was going on. The realization that I had been in surgery for 23.5 hours made it clear to me that things had not gone as planned.

The surgeons came by to visit with me. My wife and my mother were standing by, and they tried to be encouraging. Yet I could tell that they were concerned. Their greatest concern was about my eyes rolling around. They kept checking my vision with lights, holding up fingers, and asking me to concentrate on something.

Everything was exhausting. I felt I was in a race for my survival. At times, I got frustrated, not being able to move or have control over my body. I got frustrated trying to determine what was real and what was not.

The dreams continued to plague me. I dreamed that I was watching surgery from outside myself, or that I had died in surgery. When I would communicate this, I didn't feel like I was being taken seriously.

Dave, who worked the day shift, was partly responsible for my recovery. The swing shift and night shift nurses just concentrated on my care, but Dave would talk to me and get me up. He would have the other nurses help him. They would grab the sheets, pick me up, and put me in the chair and prop me up.

At first this was so tiring I would fall asleep right there in the chair. Everything would start spinning, and I would start throwing up. They would have to come in and grab me and suction me so that nothing would get into my lungs. I felt very vulnerable, as if I could die any time.

Dave kept telling me I needed to keep up the fight.

I would fall asleep and dream that I was better and could get up and walk. Then I would wake up and I was still the same. The staff told about certain signs they were looking for, but I was still thinking that to get out of ICU, I needed to walk out.

They wanted me to keep fighting so that I could leave, I had already been there longer than they expected.

I really tried. It took all my strength to move my right arm, or talk, or try to focus on something. I would fall asleep even after a short conversation, but never for long.

One day, Dave came in to check me over and talk to me like he always did. He held up his hand and said, "Try to hit my hand." So I threw a punch and hit it! He got excited and said, "All right, you are on your way out of here."

I wondered why they were transferring me out of ICU. I wasn't walking, I couldn't communicate, I was hardly able to move. I panicked.

CHAPTER 11

Very shortly the staff came to move me. Everyone was excited. My wife was trying to be excited for me. My mother was excited and telling me about the room I would be moving to with bars above the bed. It was a big day, but I felt I wasn't ready yet.

That morning they came for me with a gurney. Dave encouraged me by saying that I would be getting better, he told me to keep up the fight.

To be honest, I was very worried, but they put me on a gurney and wheeled me up to my new room on the eighth floor. This room was a little bigger, but it didn't have all the equipment of ICU. Someone showed me the view from my window of the freeway I used to take to work everyday I was exhausted from the move and must have slept for quite awhile. When I woke up, the night nurse was on duty. My wife and my mother were there, and I asked them what had happened. To me, it seemed that it should be daylight. The last thing I remember was staring at the freeway I used to take to work, and now it was dark. I tried to talk. It was hard. I couldn't speak very loudly yet. I had to whisper, and people had a hard time understanding me.

I decided I didn't want to struggle anymore.

I was tired of fighting. I was using all my strength just to get better. I wanted to be on life support. I thought they could hook me to some machines and put me out until I got better.

No one could understand what I wanted, so someone got me a pencil. Using the back of a Kleenex box I managed, after several tries, to scratch out the words "life support."

My wife said, "Do you want life support?" and I gestured with my hand, *yes*.

She looked at me and smiled. "Honey, life support is for people who can't do anything for themselves."

I thought that I couldn't do anything for myself, but she reminded me that I could breathe by myself and I was getting better.

I couldn't see it. Almost 24 hours in surgery was a long time. I thought everyone was just telling me I would get better to humor me, and they weren't being honest with me.

I didn't notice it, but as the days went by, I was able to talk better. I still wasn't eating. I lived on cranberry juice and Sustacal.

One aide named Sheila came in and talked to me about the Lord. She told me she would keep praying for me.

The days were hard, because there was a lot of activity. The physical therapist and the occupational therapist would come in and try to get me to move. Gradually my arm started coming back. My right leg was very swollen, yet my left leg was the side that was most affected. I couldn't move my legs, and I had little control over my left arm. I could move it, but it would shake and wander all over the place. The occupational therapist worked with my hands and gave me putty to squeeze. Despite all the exercises, I couldn't see any big improvements, yet I was trying so hard.

When the physical therapists came in, they would sit me up and try to teach me to hold myself up. While they held me up, they would rock me back and forth to help strengthen my trunk. I wanted to try and sit up by myself, and I did for a few seconds. Then I fell over and hit my head on the bar across the foot of my bed. The therapists were concerned, but I told them that it was the side of my head that was numb anyway, and they started to laugh.

Sheila and the rest of the staff continued to encourage me and was trying to get me to eat. Daytimes were very strenuous with blood tests and therapy, but the nights were difficult, because I had dreams all night.

One night I dreamed that the apartment below our house was on fire. I was crawling along the floor with my kids while the smoke poured from the vents. I started banging on the floor, trying to get the attention of the family that lived downstairs. They wouldn't wake up. I was panicking. Everyone was going to perish and I wouldn't be able to save them because I couldn't walk.

I woke up terrified. When the nurse asked what was wrong, I told her my house was on fire and I needed to see my wife.

She told me it was just a dream. I got angry, because I believed it really had happened. When I saw my wife, I asked her if the house was okay. She told me it was. I told her to check all the smoke detectors. She reassured me that it was all taken care of.

Another time I had a dream that I was in a small town. Terrorists had invaded the town and were shooting everybody on sight. There was panic, and I was running through the streets trying to avoid them. I ran out of an alleyway and came upon a terrorist.

He spun around with his gun and smiled at me.

I told him, "Please sir, don't shoot me."

To my relief he told me that he wouldn't shoot me. Then he said the guy behind me was going to shoot me. I spun around, he shot me in the stomach and I fell.

In my dream I pretended I was dead. After they walked off, I got up and ran out of town.

I was in the woods, running as fast as I could. I ran down

a path while the blood poured from my wound. I decided to get off the path so they couldn't find me. I ran over logs and through the heavy brush, all the while getting weaker and weaker. Finally, I jumped over an old, half-rotten log and hid inside. I was looking up to the sky as I lay dying, and I started praying the Lord's prayer.

In my dream I could feel the life draining out of me. Again I woke up terrified. I told the nurse I was dying. I had been shot. She reassured me that it was just a bad dream.

Whenever I came out of my dreams, it was so hard to come back to reality. I would think, *They are just dreams, but they seemed so real.* The dreams continued, and every day was a battle. Sometimes my dad came, and he would sit by my bed. Having him beside me, I was finally able to sleep for longer periods of time.

On Mother's Day, Sheila came in. I was feeling bad that I couldn't give my mom a Mother's Day present. I was disoriented when I first woke up and I thought she was my mother for a minute. She said she was flattered. Sheila talked about her son and told me not to worry about not being able to get my mom a present, I should just concentrate on getting well.

One of the night nurses was unkind to me. When I would call for a nurse after waking from a bad dream sometimes he would ignore my call light. Or he would come in to my room irritated and would just want me to take more pills. I couldn't really tell what kind of pills he was giving me. In my confusion I was afraid he was giving me a new medicine that is used on the mentally ill to paralyze them or put them into a coma. He wouldn't talk to me. He would just give me pills, shut off the light, and leave the room.

By then I could yell a little bit, so I would yell, and I thought I could hear him sometimes, outside the door laughing at me. I would fight going to sleep. It was like trying to fight dying. I would grab for the phone, to call for help, but it was disconnected. Then, I would start fading out because of the pills and in my panic, I knocked the phone off the night stand.

This happened more than once. Very early one morning this same night nurse came in and said something to me. I tried to respond, but I was afraid of him. He walked over to the sink and looked in the mirror to fix his hair—and I know this was real—he said that they should drug me up and forget about me. It would be easier on everybody.

When my mom came that morning, I told her that my phone had been unplugged and I couldn't call anyone. I told her what the nurse had said to me. She got very upset. She called the day nurse in and told her.

The day nurse said, "Well, I'll take care of that." My wife told me later that he had been taken off my case and was no longer allowed to come to my room. That made me feel safer.

I was still fighting, but I was tired. I was frustrated because of the dreams and because I felt I wasn't making any real progress.

Dr. Tanabe had been coming in almost every day to talk to me. He would tell me I needed to eat and he wanted me to be able to go without a catheter. Finally, one Friday, he said, "I'm going to have to tube feed you after the week end because you are still not eating."

That Sunday I prayed and told God that I had had enough. I had been here for almost a month and I was tired of fighting. I couldn't fight any more, and I wanted to die. I couldn't keep it up since I wasn't getting better. I didn't want to live this way. Even though I was able to move my arms and I was able to talk, it still wasn't much of a life. I told the Lord it was time to take me Home, and I asked Him to take care of my family.

To my surprise, I heard the voice of God speak clearly to me in my mind and heart. He said, "Tomorrow you will walk." I had never heard God talk to me like that before. I had lived an unfaithful life. I felt like I didn't deserve His help. Even though I was sure I had heard Him say I would walk, I didn't believe anything would really happen. After-all, I couldn't eat, go to the bathroom or even sit up besides not being able to walk. It seemed impossible to me so I started to doubt what I had heard.

My mom came to see me the next morning. I told her what I had heard and I asked her, " Do you think that was God?" She said very simply, "Yes, I think that was God."

When Dr. Tanabe came in on his rounds. He told me he was going to take the catheter out and I would have to go to the bathroom. He said it like there just weren't any other options. He took the catheter out himself, which was unusual. Usually neurosurgeons don't! He said in a serious voice, "You have to go." He meant no more fooling around.

Then I told him that I was going to walk today. He looked at me and said "Well, if you go to the bathroom that'll be good enough," He handed me the urinal and left.

After trying for an hour I finally went. I got so excited about my accomplishment I buzzed the nurse repeatedly. She came running in, thinking it was an emergency, and asked me what was wrong. I told her, "I went to the bathroom."

She said, "Honey, that's not an emergency."

I said, "When it's been as long as it has been for me, it is."

She laughed.

That afternoon, my wife had just left to go down to the lobby to buy gifts for the nurses when the physical therapists walked in and asked me, "Well, Rick what are you going to do today?"

I told them I was going to walk.

They said, "Why don't we try sitting up first."

They sat me up on the edge of the bed and did the usual rocking me back and forth to build up my trunk strength. All of a sudden, I felt this huge burst of energy come through my body, and I told them I was going to walk.

They just stood there looking at me. Then I stood up.

I think they finally realized I wasn't kidding.

They scrambled around and got the walker and put it in front of me, and I grabbed onto it. I wasn't graceful, but I started walking. I took off out the door and started walking down the hallway. I looked like a toddler taking his first steps. The therapists were following me, saying, "Good job! That's great! I can't believe it. That's wonderful. That's amazing!"

At the end of the hall, they brought a wheelchair, because I got really tired. I had walked about fifty feet, which was incredible. They hadn't expected me to walk for a long time if ever. They put me in a wheelchair, wheeled me over by the nurse's station and told me to sit there while they did their paper-work. I began talking to the guy who was the receptionist, and we were cracking jokes. He told me it was about time I got out of that room. Then everybody got busy doing what they normally do.

I wanted to see my wife. So I took off. I managed to wheel away without anyone seeing me. I rolled down the hall to the elevators and wheeled myself against the wall. I sat there hoping she would come up.

After I sat there for about fifteen minutes, I started getting sick. My equilibrium was still very damaged, and it was hard for me to sit up for long periods of time. I was getting nauseous, so I wheeled myself back into my room.

The nurse said, "Oh, there you are. Let's get you back into bed."

I told her, "No." I asked her to roll me over to the sink so I could throw up. She said I needed to get back in bed, and I told her, "No, not until my wife sees me!" I sat in my wheelchair up against the wall, while she ran out and paged my wife. My wife came up immediately. She walked in, and I was sitting there. She got very excited and came over and threw her arms around me.

When I told her that I had walked, she became very, very excited. I told her, "Lets go for a ride."

She wheeled me out in the hall to the observation room, which overlooked the city. Just as we went by the elevators, my uncle came off the elevator. He said, "Rick!"

I said, "Bill," and we started laughing.

He said, "You're up!" and I had my wife tell him what had happened. Was he excited! And no wonder. The last time he saw me I could barely talk.

We looked over the city for awhile and then, I got tired, so I asked them to take me back to my room. The nurses helped me get back into bed.

That was the beginning. It was the point where I finally let go and realized I couldn't do it anymore. I was in God's hands.

I had always thought that if I fought a little harder, or worked a little harder, things would get better. But I was starting to see that even though there were a lot of things I couldn't control, God was in control and He does what He says He will do. This was a turning point for me. After that, I started improving much faster than the doctors anticipated.

CHAPTER 12

The day that I walked, Dr. Tanabe came in later that afternoon. He hadn't spoken to the nurses yet, but he asked me if I had gone to the bathroom. I told him, yes, four times, and I had also walked. He threw a cheer. He thrust his arm in the air and said, "Hooray!" It was neat to watch this highly revered professional acting like a cheerleader. He told me I was on my way to Providence Hospital for rehabilitation.

I started eating soft foods like mashed potatoes and cream of wheat, but it was very tiring. I would eat for five minutes; then I would have to go to sleep. It was amazing. Something that we take for granted, like eating a hamburger, was impossible for me.

My mother would come in the morning before work and then again in the evening to feed me. She had a lot more time than the nurses, who had a hectic schedule. They were always in a hurry.

When my wife was there, she would feed me. Then, suddenly, I started noticing that although she had been there for a time following the surgery, she wasn't coming around as much.

One lunch time the nurses were in a big hurry. They were trying to feed me fast, and I couldn't handle having the food just shoved down, so I managed to call my wife. She wasn't home, so I left a message on the answering machine.

Out of my frustration I said, "You need to come up here. They don't know how to feed me. I don't understand why you haven't been coming."

After that she didn't come see me for three days. I remember calling but she was either not home or wasn't answering. I would leave messages and ask her where she was and why she wasn't coming. Finally she came to see me. All she could say was that she had been busy. She seemed different to me. I noticed that she was all dressed up and was wearing a lot of make-up. She didn't stay very long.

Therapy was very exhausting. Everyday the therapists would have me stand up and walk in the parallel bars. Then there would be a lot of other strengthening exercises to do as well.

One time my dad and my step-mom came to watch me. The therapists had me sit on a bench. I was moving a giant rubber ball around with my hands.

Then one of the therapist said, "Okay, now close your eyes and do it." So I closed my eyes and moved the ball around with my hands. It was difficult, and I just sat there.

Then the therapist asked me if I was okay. I told her, "Yes, be quiet. I'm using the force." They all laughed. I noticed my sense of humor was coming back.

One of the therapists was a petite redhead. She had a serious look on her face all the time. The other therapist was named Kelly. One time Kelly came up by herself to do my therapy, and I asked her "Where's the other one?" She asked which one and I said, "The redhead. You know, the mean one."

Kelly laughed and said she was going to tell her what I had said. The next time I saw the redhead, she said to me "I heard you think I'm mean." She laughed and told me, "You'll think meanness once you get over to Providence to the rehab ward. Now they are mean!"

I kept wondering why my wife wouldn't come. I knew my relatives were in town. She told me she needed to deal with the kids, because she had been with me for so many days straight. I knew she could find baby-sitters and that friends had offered to watch them. I sensed something was wrong, but I couldn't concentrate on it.

My mom and my older brother, Thom, visited me on a regular basis. These were the two people who had suffered the most from my marriage. My wife had convinced me in the past that my brother Thom was a opportunist and cared about me only when he needed something.

My brother would visit me at night every time I asked him, even though this was difficult for him with a wife and new baby. His wife was in school, and he worked hard as a mechanic all day. Still, he would come and read the Bible to me; or just sit and talk.

I remembered how one time before I had walked, the nurse had to change my bed and had decided to see if I could sit in a wheelchair. With my brother's help, I was able to sit. Halfway through the bed changing, I suddenly became sick. Thom wheeled me over to the sink, I didn't have the strength to hold my head up, so Thom held my head while I threw up.

No matter how unpleasant the situation, he was there to hold me up. He really showed me love. How could I have been so wrong about him? I decided then I would never let anything come between us again.

Finally Dr. Tanabe told me that I was being released from the hospital. They were going to send me to Providence Hospital's rehabilitation ward. I had mixed emotions. I was looking forward to it. Even though I was making good progress, it seemed so slow. I wanted to be better quicker. I was ready to leave behind being an invalid but I wondered if I was going to get better or not. Would I ever be the same again? I guess only God knew what my future was.

CHAPTER 13

The day for me to leave St. Vincent's Hospital was here. A man who specialized in rehabilitation came and evaluated me.

Dr. Tanabe signed my discharge papers and talked to the guy from Providence about my surgery; how difficult it was, and how long it took. He told him how happy he was that I was making enough progress to be leaving. He had been worried about me. My doctors had been unsure how much I would recover.

Dr. Tanabe told him I was a real fighter, one of the toughest guys he had seen in a long time. Funny, I didn't feel tough. In fact, I felt very vulnerable. My whole life I had been known as a hard worker and physically tough. Now, I was at the mercy of everyone else. I really couldn't have defended myself if I'd had to. That was very frustrating for me.

I also had lost half of my face. That made me feel unattractive. I had never considered myself a Hollywood pretty boy, but I was fairly handsome. Basically, I was stripped of everything a man identifies with. I was stripped of my physical abilities, I was stripped of my ability to work. I was stripped of my ability to take care of my wife.

Suzanne, the head nurse on the day shift, came in to say goodbye. She had taken good care of me and I felt a special attachment to her. It was a very hot day so the staff got me dressed in my shorts.

My wife was there with a video camera. My children and my mother were there, and it was like a celebration. It was exciting. My son had brought me a baseball cap to wear, and I put my hat and shoes on. When the transport van arrived, they put me in a wheelchair.

All the nurses told me, "Good-bye," and "Good Luck," and "You're going to do just fine."

As they took me down the hall, my wife was filming me, and my oldest son was pushing my wheelchair. I was actually sad. I had formed attachments to that room and these staff members. When people take care of your every need, you feel close to them.

Now I was leaving; going out in the world. I experienced a keen sense of loss. I was going to miss them.

As I was being wheeled through the lobby, I was sure everyone was staring at me; trying to figure out what was wrong with me. Whenever I had seen someone in a wheelchair, or someone who didn't look normal, I would wonder what had happened to that person. Now I was the one in a wheelchair who didn't look normal. I was the one someone would be wondering about. I felt very self-conscious.

The people from transport loaded me on the van. My oldest son got to ride with us. They put me on a lift, raised my chair and strapped me down. My wife and my mom followed in another car.

My son thought the ride was great. It was hot, but the van was air conditioned. It was a difficult ride for me. The movement of the van affected my equilibrium. I felt sick, and tried to hold myself, so I wouldn't move around too much. Luckily, the ride was short.

Providence Hospital was different. My room was farther away from the nurses' station and a different color. My wife was still filming me as I got into bed and took off my shoes. The nurse checked me in and told me all about the ward. They asked me questions, such as: What day is it? What is your name? Where do you live? How many fingers am I holding up?

By the time I was all checked in, I was exhausted. I fell asleep. When I woke up, my wife wasn't there. I remember her telling me she would leave as soon as I fell asleep. The nurse told me the physical therapist would come in soon and talk to me. When the therapist came in she told me they would be working on setting up a routine was so I could take care of myself and learn to meet my own needs. It was a big step.

My first day at Providence I was evaluated by Dr. Anderson; a rehabilitation specialist. I told him I hadn't had a real shower since my operation, so he told me he would make arrangements. That night I got a shower sitting on a shower stool and accompanied by a nurse's aid.

The next day was a new beginning. The staff came in and gave me my schedule. They asked me questions again about what my name was, where I lived, and what day it was.

I found myself getting irritated. I could still think fairly clearly, but physically my body wasn't responding and doing what I told it to do. My thinking capacity was fine, but the pathways that carried the messages were scrambled.

This is why surgery on the brain stem is difficult to predict. I had some damage where they cut the cerebellum. Any trauma to the brain will affect your thinking, especially when you are tired. I felt like some of the staff was talking to me like I was a child. I wondered why they kept asking me the same questions they had asked me the day before.

A speech therapist came in. She took me to the cafeteria to watch me eat. Before I came to Providence, I had eaten a chicken enchilada which was very good. I knew I could eat solid food, but I had to be careful because I had bitten my tongue a few times.

I told her I could eat solid food. She took the cover off the plate and it was pureed. It was green. I looked at her.

"This is pureed food," I said. " I told you I could eat solid food."

She said they were worried and had to see for themselves. I asked her what the food was. She looked at it and admitted she didn't know.

"If you don't even know what it is, I sure am not going to eat it. Get me some solid food!" I demanded.

It took a little while but she got me some chicken and dumplings. She sat, watching me while I ate, and I did okay. I had to open up my mouth after I was done, to make sure there was no food caught in my left cheek. Every once in while I would bite my tongue on the side where I didn't have any feeling, but so far I hadn't choked or aspirated anything into my lungs.

Next, an occupational therapist came in and evaluated me. She tested my grip strength and my steadiness. After that I went to Physical Therapy where I was tested on my standing and walking abilities. I also did various balance exercises. The staff had me stand with a walker, because I couldn't stand unassisted yet. They had me close my eyes. As soon as I closed my eyes, I fell over. My balance was still affected.

One of the assistants named David was an intern. He had graduated from his physical therapy course, but he had one more year as an intern before he could get his license. He would be doing a lot of my 'hands on' personal therapy. The main therapists would set up what they wanted to accomplish, and he would do it.

I practiced walking. I was told to concentrate on not walking with such a wide stance. They would hold me up and throw a ball at me and have me try and kick it. I was learning very fast.

My mother still came every morning and evening. My wife wasn't coming to see me much. When I asked her to come, she told me it was really quite impossible, because she had to deal with the kids, who needed her. I had been at Providence for three days and she hadn't been there since the first day.

Every day was filled with physical therapy. The head therapist's name was Jean, and she was pretty tough. We liked to joke back and forth and talk about wrestling and cookies. I told her I would bring her a cookie if she would take it easy on me. She would just laugh and say, "Not on your life."

The therapists were happy with my progress. Soon, I could walk much more for longer periods with the walker. I could walk without the walker, but they didn't want me to, because I walked very stiff legged and it wasn't good for me.

It was important how I relearned to walk.

My schedule was very rigorous. I went to occupational therapy, then physical therapy. I would eat lunch, then go to occupational therapy, then physical therapy again. In between I would do recreational therapy where we would do things like sit in chairs and do rhythmic arm movements to music.

The occupational therapist came in the mornings and laid out my clothes. She would tell me I had five minutes to get dressed and leave. After physical therapy I would go back to my room and fall asleep which would make me late to the rec-room for occupational therapy, and the therapist would come to my room and scold me. Between not falling asleep at night and the demands of my therapy schedule, most of the time I was exhausted.

I had been taught to get into my wheelchair and go to the bathroom by myself but I was not allowed to do it without a nurse there to watch me. I was frustrated, because when I rang for the nurse to use the bathroom, it would sometimes take someone a half an hour to get there. They got irritated with me when one time I couldn't wait so I went by myself. I told them I couldn't always hold it for a half hour and besides it was degrading to me to have a nurse watch me go.

Every morning the nurses still asked me what my name was, where I lived, and what day it was. One morning I got upset and asked them why they asked me the same question every morning. I told them they should write it down so they wouldn't forget and have to keep coming in and asking me the same thing. I was sorry to be sarcastic, but it was my way of telling them I was getting tired of them asking me the same questions every morning. They got the hint, I guess, because after that they stopped.

When I talked to Dr. Rohrer about how I felt, he told me the nurses weren't used to cases like mine, where the higher functions were still there, even though I was physically limited. Mostly, they worked with stroke patients and severe head injuries, who had lost most of their cognitive abilities.

This information helped a little with my frustration. I could see the nurses weren't used to people like me; they were doing the best they could.

I had told some of the night nurses that my surgery had taken almost 24 hours, and after I had gotten out of surgery things looked pretty bad for a while and my doctors were worried I wasn't going to recover. I told them about how I had heard from God and walked the next day and that I had been making great progress ever since. They would say, "Oh, that's great." I could see they didn't really know how to respond. It seemed odd when I told them something that was amazing to me, yet they didn't know what to say. I realized that I just couldn't talk to anyone and expect them to believe.

My wife finally had come a couple of times, but there

would be a three day stretch between visits. She would come and complain that she didn't like me being in the hospital; she didn't think I was getting good enough care and she wanted me to come home. That didn't make sense to me because she wasn't visiting me that often. I wondered how my kids were doing. I hadn't seen them but a few times since my surgery.

My brother, Steve, came to visit and brought pizza. It was the first time I had had pizza since my surgery. It was difficult to eat, but I forced myself. It tasted wonderful.

I still had a pressure sore on my chest. All of a sudden, it became numb. Dr. Tanabe had one of his associates examine it. He told me the scar tissue had affected the nerves and it was nothing to be alarmed about.

Dr. Canepa came to see me hoping I had made up my mind about the nerve graft.

Melanie still had her doubts.

Finally, I said, "Let's do the surgery." He asked me if I was sure and if my wife was OK with my decision. I told him, "It's my face. It has to be my decision. I can't sit here and let everyone argue about this anymore. I've made up my mind. I want the surgery. Let's do it."

CHAPTER 14

Dr. Canepa set the date for my next surgery which was only about a week away. I went for ultrasounds on my legs to see if I had blood clots. They found a blood clot in my left leg; it was small, so it wasn't considered threatening. I had to have it checked every day until my surgery, because they couldn't put me on blood thinners with the surgery coming up.

I had a lot of fear. Dr. Canepa told me the surgery would take four to six hours. I had been told my first surgery would take eight to twelve hours, yet I was in there for almost twenty-four hours and I came out a lot worse than I had expected. I couldn't help having a lot of anxiety. My wife accepted my decision to have the surgery, and that helped.

While I was at Providence, Dr. Anderson was in charge of my case. Once a day, he would come in to talk to me, ask how I was doing, and if I needed anything. I told him my wife really wanted me to come home. I was tired of being in the hospital. I wanted to get home as fast as I could.

Dr. Anderson told me I was making faster progress than

expected. He offered me a weekend pass to see how I would do.

My mom, my wife, and my brothers arranged for a picnic. They came and got me on Saturday. I was still fighting fatigue and the car ride to the park wore me out. Someone put up a lawn chair for me and I took a nap; then we ate. My kids wanted to go to the river, so my brother wheeled me down to the river and I watched my kids play.

The rest rooms were not wheelchair accessible. They were outhouses so my brother had to help me up. It was embarrassing. A lot of your dignity is taken away when you have to let someone help you to the bathroom.

The picnic went pretty well. We stayed all day and packed up in the evening. My wife took me back to the hospital.

The next day I got a pass and went home. I rested and visited with my kids. My wife told me how nice it was to have me home. We talked about my surgery and how hard it had been on her. It was hard to be in my house, because I was not the same person as before.

I realized I was still short tempered, easily frustrated, and my emotions were hard to control. Going into surgery I had thought it would change me, and take away my problems, but in many ways I was worse off. I felt it wasn't fair that I had to go through all this and still struggle with myself. I realized that even a dramatic surgery like mine couldn't change me. I had to work at it and take steps to change.

I stayed up for quite a while and it got very late. My wife called the hospital and told them I was too tired and had overdone it that day. So, I got to sleep in my own bed again next to my wife. It felt strange but nice. The next day, my wife took me back to the hospital. She told me she didn't like it there; she thought I could do just fine at home.

I discussed this with Dr. Anderson who was reluctant to discharge me. They were concerned, because I was pushing it awfully hard. He said if I was too impatient to wait for the nurses he was afraid that I wouldn't use good judgment at home. But I felt I knew within myself what my limitations were. The doctor agreed to look into my leaving the hospital and said the staff would hold a meeting. I agreed to leave the decision up to him.

The dust had settled and I started feeling lonely. I was going to be okay. I was far from recovered, but I was making progress. The big emergency was over, so except for my mom, I didn't have many visitors.

I continued with therapy. It became harder. The staff kept pushing me. I began thinking that no one really understood what I was going through, or how hard it was to learn to walk all over again. How much we take for granted! Simple things, such as brushing our teeth, getting up, going to the bathroom, walking and eating without difficulty.

Mealtimes were a challenge for me. I went down the hall to eat. When I ate, I wouldn't talk to anyone, because it was hard for me to eat with half of my face paralyzed. I had to concentrate.

I was sitting there one time when a visitor sat down across from me. He looked over at me and sarcastically asked what a young guy like me was doing there with all these mature people. I looked at him and said, "I'm eating." He told me it looked good and I told him. "It is. Now leave me alone, so I can finish."

I'm not usually that way, but after my surgery I didn't have much tolerance for people who didn't realize how much of a challenge it was to eat without spilling food all over myself. Realistically I couldn't expect him to understand. But I didn't have the time or energy to be diplomatic, so I was blunt.

The days drifted by, and finally Dr. Canepa, my plastic surgeon, came in and reaffirmed my next surgery. Shortly after that, Dr. Anderson told me they had agreed to release me to go home. He said there wasn't much point keeping me when I didn't want to be there, and he thought I would be all right at home. I would be released on Wednesday and go into surgery on Thursday. I thought, *Oh boy, I get to go home for one day before I go back to surgery.*

I called my wife the day before my release to come pick

me up. She said she planned to go to a parade with the kids and suggested I find someone else to come get me.

I told her it was okay, but deep down I was hurt. I couldn't believe it at first because she had told me how she wanted me to come home. It just didn't make sense.

All of a sudden, it seemed it didn't really matter to her. I had hoped we would make a big deal out of it. We would go home together and have a good time with the kids and just enjoy the moment. It should have been a big celebration.

I was hurt and confused, also scared about the upcoming surgery. After my last surgery, I was a little gun shy.

I called my brother Steve and he came and got me the next day. He took me home and my wife arrived shortly after I got there. The kids were happy to see me. The house was a mess, and my wife was stressed out. She finally told me she was happy to see me. We hung out, talked to the kids, and I got tired and went to bed early.

CHAPTER 15

My wife and I arrived at St. Vincent's Hospital at eleven the next day. We checked in and went through the same routine. I was wheeled up to the pre-surgical floor. The nurse took my blood pressure, hooked up my IV, and asked me the same old questions.

Shortly after, someone came and put me on the gurney. I looked up and it was Bob, the same guy who taken me to my first surgery. It was nice to see a familiar face. He wheeled me into the same room I had before my brain surgery. Memories came rushing back. It was a very sobering moment. I started experiencing some of the same fears. I couldn't believe that I was in the same room with the same nurses, who remembered me. It was spooky.

My wife held my hand. We had arranged to have the same anesthesiologist, Dr. Evans. He came in and was glad to see me. He gave me some medication to help me relax.

I think I was more scared this time than before my first

surgery. When it came time to go, I said good-bye to my wife once again.

They wheeled me into the operating room, and it was as cold as I remembered. It was like returning to the scene of the crime. It was cold, scary, and sterile. I started having flashbacks. The last time I was here, my whole life changed. What would happen to me now?

The table in the operating room was different. It was a soft table this time. Dr. Canepa came in with Dr. Evans, and I just stared at them. They could see from the look in my eyes, how scared I was. Dr. Canepa grabbed my hand and told me it would be okay.

Then, Dr. Evans, the anesthesiologist, told me, "Okay, I am going to put you out now." As I fell down the black hole the light got smaller and smaller and then *boom,* I was out.

I woke up in the post-op ward. Dr. Canepa was there looking me over. They knew I would wake up fighting so they had me tied down as a safeguard. I did wake up scared, disoriented, and thrashing around. Dr. Evans came over and gave me something to calm me down. They wheeled me up to a room on the same floor. It was late at night. My wife told me the surgery took eight hours instead of six. I thought, *Oh no. Not again.*

When I became alert, my mom and my wife were there. I looked like I had been hit by a truck, then dumped into a meat grinder. I had an incision on my right leg that started halfway up my calf and ran all the way past my ankle to my foot. I had an incision on the side of my face that ran from the top of my head all the way down past my ear, curved around, and went halfway across my neck. I had another incision in the middle of my lip and one right in between my eyes.

My wife was looking me over. She pushed me over on my side and looked under my right knee, where they had made the incision.

All of a sudden she exclaimed, "Oh my God! They didn't suture this incision."

She ran out to the nurse's station and the nurses came in. They looked at my wife in disbelief. The incision was about an inch long open, gaping wound.

My wife got upset and told them to call Dr. Canepa at home. The nurse called him from my room and told us the doctor said to pack it with gauze.

My wife said, " No way!"

She got the doctor on the phone, and he repeated the order, "Just pack it with gauze. It will be okay."

My wife hung up, but she started getting more and more upset. She went to the nurse's station and got the head nurse.

Melanie told her, "Look, my husband just went through eight hours of surgery, and they forgot to suture an incision. I want this sewed up now!"

Things were riled up around there. It got late so my wife left. My mom stayed.

Around midnight Dr. Canepa came by in a sweatshirt and jeans. He told us he couldn't sleep, knowing he had forgotten an incision. He pulled out a small kit, numbed the area, and just sewed it up. He apologized to my mother and told us he was sorry for the mistake.

Dr. Canepa was very humble. He told us there were many incisions for this surgery. In concentrating on the nerves in my face, he had overlooked the incision on my leg.

The next day was Friday. I had been sick all day. My wife brought the kids up. I was worried about the kids, because the bandages had just been removed. I looked pretty bad. I had a lot of stitches. The kids stopped at the doorway, stared at me, then proceeded very slowly into the room.

They adjusted quickly. "What's that on your face, Dad?" they asked. "Boy, they really cut you up this time, Dad."

Mallory, my four year old, wanted to sit on the bed. Then they wanted to watch TV and run around the room.

I looked at my wife to communicate that it was getting late, and the kids were getting rambunctious. It seemed to me that she didn't want to be there anyway. I asked her if she would come see me the next day, She told me she didn't know. She wanted to do yard work and get some work done around the house. I felt hurt but, of course, I told her okay.

The next morning I was very sick, so I called my wife, and she said she would try to come, but she was busy with kids.

I was in a lot of pain. Every time I threw up, it felt like my face was tearing apart. I discovered when you throw up, you tense your whole body because even the stitches on my legs hurt.

There I was alone. The nurse did a good job of caring for me, but she was busy. I thought my stomach was empty, yet I filled the pan up so it spilled on my bed. It was horrible. I can't ever remember being in greater agony, except for the time when I was in ICU.

This time I was more alert, and it was a different kind of pain. I could feel the nausea building, and I would think, *Oh my God, here I go again!* Every time I threw up it felt like all my stitches were splitting open. My face was swollen. I had to keep the vomit out of my stitches because of the risk of infection. I couldn't believe this was happening to me.

This was supposed to be a simple operation, yet it was the third day and I was still sick. I wondered why I had to go through it alone. I called my wife again and got the answering machine.

The day went on and the nurses called the doctor. He thought maybe the painkiller was making me sick, so they stopped it, but it didn't help. Then he decided it might be caused by the antibiotic, but he didn't want to discontinue it, so I had to put up with being sick all day long. In the evening the antibiotic was stopped. After a couple hours my stomach settled down, so it must have been the antibiotic.

Finally, my wife showed up in the evening. A little late. My brother came up, too. I could have called my mother or my brother earlier. I love them, but I felt a wife should support her husband in times of trouble. Her attitude had me confused.

During the first surgery my wife and I were close. I took it for granted she would be there for me, but now everything had changed. I felt like I didn't fit into her life anymore.

She visited for awhile, but I was exhausted. I had been in a race all day against the nausea.

Sunday came. Dr. Webber, another plastic surgeon, came by and told me they would discontinue the Motrin. He asked me if I had pain in my legs. I told him no, and he thought that was rare. I had a lot of pain in my face. Dr. Webber told me I could go home on Monday. My nausea was under control, and my stitches were fine. My mom came to visit me and my brother, but my wife did not.

I called my wife to tell her I would be released from the hospital on Monday morning. She said she had to take the kids to school and do errands, and it would be hard for her to come pick me up. I couldn't believe what I was hearing. She didn't work. The two boys went to school, and I would be discharged about noon. Obviously she didn't want to pick me up.

So I called my mom, who works, and she told me, "Sure, I'll come get you." She arranged to come at noon and took a long lunch.

The nurse helped me take a shower. I was so filthy. Just my luck, the shower wasn't working right and I kept getting shocks of cold water. She felt bad about it after all I had been through. She had taken care of me after my first surgery, too. The shower just wouldn't cooperate. It was all we could do to get me washed up without freezing to death.

But we got through it and laughed a little.

Then my mom arrived to take me home.

CHAPTER 16

I was finally home. My kids were happy to see me, but my wife was stressed. She was trying to do the best she could. She had set up a bed and she brought me juice, but she didn't come in to sit with me and talk to me. I felt alone, emotionally abandoned. This was not what I had in mind.

The kids came in, but my wife kept busy. She seemed to resent the added responsibility. Now she not only had the kids to deal with, but I was home and needing care.

My problems were still very real, my temper was worse. When I got stressed out or tired, I felt pressure in my head. I would snap easily and was less able to deal with things. I had thought I would come out of surgery and be a more peaceful man with a greater perspective on life. I did have a different perspective, but there was a lot of damage and swelling after surgery and I felt hostile, sensing that things had changed with my wife.

The distance between us was growing greater. She

seemed disappointed the way things had turned out. I sensed she was struggling, torn between what she wanted to do and what she thought she had to do. It was amazing, through all the trauma that was done to me, I was still perceptive.

Still, I was tired and couldn't think very well. I had problems tracking conversations. I couldn't really walk; I was still in the wheelchair. I was tired all the time; I had a lot of pressure in my head, and I got dizzy spells. I still had a lot of recovery ahead of me.

My wife and I had a history of problems before my surgery. We had a poor foundation. We had married when she was on the rebound and very hurt by events in her life up to that point. Both needy, we had latched onto each other.

I had felt a strong bond existed between us that would keep us together. I had always felt she loved me before; I didn't feel that anymore. Admittedly, I was a different person physically, but my feelings and problems were the same. Only now they were amplified.

I had always been strong physically. I was very competent in handling myself. I used to box. I had taken Tai Kwan Do and Karate. I was athletic, strong, and was sure of myself. I was also a very hard worker and a fine carpenter, able to do a lot of my own remodeling. Now I wasn't capable of fixing the simplest leak under the sink. Physically, I had changed, and it was hard to accept.

I told myself, *I am not going to be this way. I am going to fight and get back on my feet and be exactly the way I was before.*

I didn't realize at the time how unrealistic that was. Now, when I came to a wall I couldn't knock down, I had to learn to go around it in a different way. I didn't have the ability anymore to knock down walls, or overcome obstacles by charging into them headlong like I used to. I was going to have to depend upon God to give me the strength and wisdom I needed to get through this.

Finally home, I didn't feel it was my home anymore. I felt like a stranger or a guest who was imposing. I felt like a burden.

The days went on about the same every day. My wife brought me my breakfast. I got into my wheelchair for awhile and observed the chaos going on. The house was a mess. My wife was stressed out, the kids were out of school and would run around the house and play all day. I slept a lot. Every day was set to the basics: Eat, sleep, and go to the bathroom.

A month went by. My wife told me we were falling behind on the bills. The money from my disability wasn't covering the mortgage. I wondered why she was telling me. I didn't feel I was in any position to deal with the bills. I was still wondering if I was ever going to get out of my wheelchair. I could walk for maybe five minutes like a toddler with my walker, and I would break out in a sweat. I was tired after eating. I just didn't understand why I was so tired all the time.

Not much attention was being paid to me. After major surgery and nearly losing my life, I had gone through yet another major surgery, I was sick. I had lost half my face and a lot of my abilities. I was trying to recover. From my viewpoint, my wife was more worried about making the mortgage payment than whether I was okay or not.

She started talking about getting a job. That scared me. I reminded her she had the kids. How was she going to get a job when I could hardly take care of myself? She said she would work graveyard. I argued that she couldn't work graveyard and get enough sleep. So she said she would work swing shift. She told me she would cook meals ahead of time. I could set the food out and monitor the kids while they got themselves ready for bed.

I told her, "These are our kids you are talking about. Even when we were both fit it was hard enough to get them to brush their teeth and go to bed. How do you expect them to do this when I am in a wheelchair most of the time?"

I suggested we sell the house. We could pay off all our debts, have some money in our pocket, rent an apartment, and live off my disability until I got back on my feet. For some reason she didn't want to do this. She wanted to get a job. I felt this was just an excuse to get away.

Before my surgery my wife had assured me we would do whatever it took to survive. We would sell the house, or even live with one of our parents so she could take care of me. Now things had changed. I felt I was low on the priority list. I felt abandoned.

CHAPTER 17

I decided that all our problems were my fault because of my surgery. I told my wife she could do whatever she wanted. Melanie immediately started looking for a job. She got very excited looking through the want ads.

Before my surgery, we hadn't had a good marriage. I hadn't been a good husband, she hadn't been a good wife and I don't think either of us had been very good parents. We had struggled and fought through most of our marriage and now I had hoped we could take advantage of this time and rebuild our family with God at the center.

She continued to take me to therapy even though it seemed like it was a hassle to her. After therapy I was always exhausted. I would have a headache and it was hard for me to sit in my wheelchair. Usually my wife was late and I would have to sit and wait. When I asked her what took so long she would tell me she had lost track of time. I felt as if she had just left me there and had forgotten about me. I would get very upset and tell her she couldn't possibly understand how hard it was for me to sit up in my wheelchair when I was worn out after therapy. She didn't seem to care. She acted like I was being unreasonable.

One weekend she told me she wanted to go to an all day country music concert. She would take me and the kids over to my mother's and then go to the concert. It was the end of June, the weather hot and I wasn't drinking as much as I was supposed to. She got back late that night and took us home. I was so exhausted that I woke up about ten a.m. the next morning. Everyone was out in the living room. I was supposed to call for help to go to the bathroom, but I looked at my walker and said to myself, *I'm going to do this myself. It's time for me to get better so I don't have to depend on everyone else.*

Since the bathroom was only one door down I thought I would just hobble in there with my walker, go to the bathroom, hobble back out and get back into bed without disturbing anyone. I got my walker and made it to the bathroom, but I started to feel sick to my stomach. The next thing I remember was waking up on the floor. I don't know how long I had been laying there passed out, but it was the strangest feeling. I didn't even remember falling. I managed to pull myself up, I still felt disoriented, and I wasn't sure where I was. I came out of the bathroom, stumbling and lightheaded, and yelled for my wife.

I made it to the bed and fell on it. She asked me what was wrong, and I told her I had passed out. I couldn't answer for a minute because the room was spinning. She got really scared. She immediately ran to the phone and called Dr. Rohrer. At first, the doctor wanted me to go to the emergency room, but I told my wife I was feeling better. I didn't want to go back to the hospital. When my wife called the doctor back to tell him I was feeling better, he asked how much I had to drink the day before. He explained to her that if people with neurological damage don't drink enough, it restricts a certain nerve and when they urinate they pass out.

My wife brought me a large glass of juice and I drank it down. She was relieved the incident was over, but it was a setback for me. Memories of being in the hospital and not having control of myself came crashing down on me. It was a horrifying experience.

Time went on and I was pushing myself to get better. I would walk around the house without my walker even though I should have been resting. I wanted to be the man I was before so I could be an important part of my wife's life again. She was preoccupied with finding a job.

My wife had applied at a pipe bending place. She didn't think she would get the job, because it was male oriented and she didn't have any experience. One day they called and asked her to come in right away. She rushed down for an interview.

She came back and said, "I can't believe it. I got the job."

She said she walked in and they asked her if she could start on July 5th. They told her what was expected of her. The position was new, an entry level job, but work was steady. That's all there was to it.

When she told me she would be on swing shift, I told her, "That's great honey."

Deep down I was very worried. She wouldn't get home until after eleven at night, and she had to get up early to take care of the kids. I knew from when I worked swing shift that it would be hard to wind down much before one in the morning. I didn't want her to burn out. I tried to be supportive even though I felt things were changing for the worse.

CHAPTER 18

On the fourth of July we were supposed to go to my mother's house with the kids. My brother, Steve, came over to go with us.

That morning I was extremely tired. My emotions for the last couple of weeks had been surging inside of me. The pressure in my head bothered me. My doctors had explained that there was still some swelling there. They warned me to be careful about getting overtired or I could become more emotional.

My wife informed me that morning that she didn't want to come with me. She wanted to stay home and clean the house but she would come that evening just in time to see the kids light their fireworks.

I started getting very upset. I said, "That's just an excuse not to be around my family, or to be with me."

Deep down, I depended on her to feel safe and take care of me, and I felt that she was the only one who understood my needs. I became extremely angry and followed her around the house. I lost control and started yelling at her. I felt like an animal being let out of a cage. I screamed that she didn't care about me. Ever since the hospital, she had tried to avoid me.

She started crying and told me she couldn't believe I was yelling at her, after all she had done for me.

I told her she had only done what she had to do. Her heart wasn't in it. My wife asked me what I was trying to say. Should we get a divorce? I didn't mean it, but I said maybe we should, and then I left with my brother.

My brother and I went up the street and bought fireworks. Then we swung back by the house. My wife's mother was there, and my wife was in tears. I tried to apologize to her and tell her that I didn't know what come over me, but she didn't want to hear it. She just wanted me to leave.

My kids and I went over to my mom's. We ate and when night fell, my wife came over, but she avoided me and just watched the kids. The next day she started her job.

That month was very tough. Melanie worked swing shift. She would get home and fall asleep around one. Then she would try to get up and take me to therapy, but sometimes I would have to take the bus home, which was very strenuous with the wheelchair.

I decided I needed to try harder to make things work. I started pushing myself to do more. I tried to let her sleep in the mornings. I even started driving the car when I wasn't supposed to. I would drive the kids to school and tried to do the laundry and dishes.

After about a week at her new job, one time Melanie didn't come home right after work. She got home around three in the morning. When I asked her where she had been, she said she had stopped at the bar for a couple drinks. The first few times this happened, I figured it was no big deal. After all, she was working hard and just wanted a couple beers after work.

Soon she started coming in late more often and she would sleep most of the day. I didn't want to cause any more waves, so I tried to do more and more around the house. Before I knew what was happening, she started coming in late every night. She would get up at one in the afternoon, just in time to go back to work. I had the kids all evening. Basically, I didn't see her anymore. I knew something was very wrong but I was in a vulnerable position, and I wanted to hang onto my marriage.

As I worked harder and harder taking care of the kids, my need for pain medication increased. I was doing more than I should, and I was in a lot of pain most of the time. I would get headaches and sore muscles.

I managed to create a schedule where the kids were helping me some. I would have dinner ready for my wife at night and pack her lunches before she went to work. I was trying to show her I was sorry, and I was making an effort to get back on my feet. I knew I wasn't in normal physical condition, but I was learning how to take care of the kids and the housework. Even though something unexpected was always coming up this was a good learning experience for me. As I got better and was doing more and more I thought she would see that we could become a peaceful family if we worked together.

CHAPTER 19

My dad called and wanted us to come visit him in Gold Beach, which is almost to the California border on the Oregon coast. I thought it would be nice for me and the kids to get away for a week. My dad came and got us at the end of August.

While we were there, it was nice because my dad and my step-mom spent a lot of time with the kids so I could rest more. I didn't have to cook or do housework. I just relaxed and enjoyed doing nothing. I realized since I had left the hospital in June, I had mostly taken care of myself and my three children and not been allowed to focus just on my recovery.

Even though I had made a miraculous recovery, I was walking more and more and gaining my strength and stamina back at a remarkable rate, I still felt robbed in some way.

We spent the week there, and towards the end of the week my Grandpa Joe and Grandma Donna came down. Grandpa

Joe was very ill. He was having problems with his lungs, and the doctors had told him he had pneumonia.

Right before we went home my Grandpa Joe gave each of the kids one hundred dollars. He said he wanted to give it to them personally, because you never know what will happen between now and Christmas. He told them it would help out with school clothes. He wanted to see the appreciation on their faces.

I got to talk to my grandpa alone, and we talked about the surgery and some personal stuff. Even though I hadn't seen him that much as I was growing up I had always felt close to him. As we talked that day, we became a little closer.

When the day came to return home, I felt hesitant. Whenever I called home I would only get Melanie occasionally. When I did catch her, she would talk to me, but I had this feeling something was going on.

Despite my misgivings, we left early in the morning because it was a seven hour drive. My dad drove, and we had to stop quite a bit with three kids. We arrived home just after nightfall.

When we came in the door, my wife had been cleaning the house frantically. This was a clue. I knew that she did this whenever she was about to drop a bomb.

Melanie hugged the kids, but she didn't seem too happy to see me. My dad left right away to get back to Gold Beach. We sat down, and the air was thick from tension in the room. I noticed my wife was smoking. She had quit ten years before, but she had started again while we were at the coast. She lit up a cigarette and stared off in the distance and blew smoke in the air, so I asked her what was up.

She said, "Well, I've been thinking while you were gone."

I looked at her, and I knew deep down what was coming. I felt like a vise was tightening around my chest. I asked her immediately if she had met someone else.

She said, "No," so we continued talking. She said, "I've been thinking, and I think I want a divorce."

I asked what brought this on. She said she didn't think there was anything left of our relationship. She wanted to find her own life and fulfill herself. The only thing I could say was, "Please, let's work this thing out. Let's go see Craig."

Craig, my counselor, had worked with both of us before. She didn't think there was anything to counsel about. She had made up her mind.

I told Melanie again, "Please, so much has happened this year. Let's give this a chance." We argued back and forth, and finally she agreed to go talk to the counselor, but she said her mind was made up. She went downstairs to sleep.

We got up the next morning, and she informed me she was put on day shift for a while. I said that was fine, because she hadn't been home anyway. She might as well work day shift. I called Craig immediately, and he agreed we could see him on Monday.

I did a lot of crying that weekend. Once again, I had something happening to me that I thought would never happen. I talked to my wife periodically and I cried and hugged her. I kept telling her I wanted to work it out and not have my kids grow up in a broken home. She would hug me back and tell me she didn't want to hurt me, but she couldn't handle things.

We went to Craig. We talked together first. Melanie told Craig she couldn't handle our relationship, and wanted to end it before she ended up hating me. I left and she talked to Craig alone. As we left she told me she had talked to Craig and that we were going to work it out.

At this point, the dam broke, and I began weeping. Melanie touched my arm and asked me what was wrong, since we were going to work it out.

I told her, "I know, but I don't want to screw it up this time. I am afraid, because I don't know what to do."

I was dealing with a lot physically and emotionally. Now I was trying to hang onto my marriage. I told her that I loved her and would do everything in my power to make sure our marriage lasted.

When we got home the kids asked why was Daddy

crying? We told them that Mommy and Daddy had some problems to work out. Things were good for about a week. I tried, but my wife didn't want to talk about anything. She really wasn't responsive. She would tell me to back off and give her space. I tried really hard to keep the house clean and pack her lunches and show her how much I cared.

I was still restricted to the wheelchair about seventy-five percent of the time. I was walking more than I was supposed to and tried to deal with the pain. I kept going to therapy and things coasted along. My wife and I would hug sometimes, but it seemed like there wasn't much feeling there. Her heart wasn't in it.

CHAPTER 20

Melanie told me how good she was doing at work and how much they appreciated her. She was getting recognition from work, and she loved the job. She also talked a lot about her boss, Mark. She told me that Mark went to counseling, because he had been divorced. She said he really understood her and could sympathize with her feelings.

One day Melanie brought home a flyer and told me there was to going to be a company picnic. I thought that was great. We got the kids ready one Saturday and we all went to the picnic. I was able to walk with a cane by this time. I talked to the owner, who had built the company with his own two hands, and I admired him for that.

I also got to meet Mark, Melanie's boss. I walked up to him and asked how he liked working with Melanie. I commented on what a good worker she was. It seemed like he didn't want to talk to me. He just said, "Yeah, she's a good one," then walked away.

The way he responded struck me as odd. Something didn't

feel right, but I just walked over to be with my family. Melanie was acting nervous. We had a good time, but I felt like a lot of people avoided us. I figured they must have felt uncomfortable around me because of my appearance.

My mother planned a weekend for me and my kids to go on a little trip to visit my aunt in Eugene, then down to the coast to see my grandmother. Melanie didn't want to go, but I thought it would be fun for the kids, so we went.

My mother and I drove on Friday with the kids to Eugene, then made our way to the Oregon coast. We spent the night in Florence and came back on Sunday. The whole time we were gone, I had the feeling something was waiting for me when we got back.

When we returned late Sunday night, I felt like I was listening to pre-recorded tape. I asked Melanie what was up. She said she had been thinking. I told her to spit it out, and she said, "I want a divorce. This isn't working."

I said she hadn't even given it a chance but she believed that it was over for her. She had too many hurts; she wanted her freedom.

I asked her about the kids. She was convinced that if it was done right, they would adjust. I didn't believe there was a right way, but there was no talking to her.

I finally realized I wasn't going to convince her. I could talk myself blue in the face, but I wasn't going to change her mind. A lot had happened in the past, but my surgery was the final straw. It was over, and there was nothing I could do about it.

I couldn't help thinking that it was poor timing. I had lost my physical well being, almost lost my life, lost my ability to work and half of my face. Everything a man identifies with, and now I was being dumped.

I felt as if I had been thrown on the ground with someone tap dancing on my head. I felt totally abandoned by someone I needed. I couldn't imagine feeling any more hurt, helpless or vulnerable.

Melanie finished her cigarette, walked in the house and went to bed.

I grabbed my cane and walked up to the bar about a block away. It was a really stupid idea, because my balance was bad, and I wasn't supposed to be walking around much with only a cane. It was the lowest time of my life; darkness surrounded me.

I drank two beers in five minutes. Then I had a third, and because of my condition, it affected me very quickly. I hadn't been drinking for about three years now. I thought to myself, *What am I doing here? I almost lost my life. I have gone through hell to get back on my feet, and now my wife is cutting out on me. Did I really go through all this to throw myself into a bottle?*

I thought about my three kids and decided I had been given a second chance in life. It would be foolish to throw it away because of her. My kids were depending on me. God must have known this was going to happen and that was why I was still here. Maybe if I give her some time she will come around .

Over the next week I observed my wife's behavior changing even more drastically. Melanie was drinking every night after work and didn't care what I thought about it.

I was home with the kids almost twenty-four hours a day. I was letting the housework slip, as my emotional state got worse.

I wasn't eating right. I was supposed to be using my face stimulator to keep my muscles toned up, and I wasn't always doing it. My health and balance were getting worse, and I was spending more time in the wheelchair. I felt like a little puppy standing on the corner of a busy intersection, lost and all alone, while the traffic whizzes by with no one paying any attention to him.

One morning I woke up to find that Melanie had already gotten up and taken the two boys to school and she had our girl with her. I got in my wheelchair and wheeled down to a nearby restaurant to get something to eat.

By the time I got home, it was time to pick the boys up from school, and I hadn't heard from her. The school was about six or seven blocks away, so I got my cane and walked down there. It was very stressful; I shouldn't have walked that far. I started getting a headache, my legs started hurting, and I was sweating profusely.

It took awhile to get there but I made it just after the bell had rang. When I went into the school Bryan's teacher told me Melanie had already picked them up. I realized she had to be at work at three-thirty and she didn't know where I was, so I tried to hurry home.

By the time I got home I was in a lot of pain. I was at the end of my rope. I came in, and she was in the bathroom putting on her makeup like she usually did before work. This had always bothered me because she went to a shop where she got greasy, sweaty and dirty. Why would she need to spend so much time on her hair and make up?

I asked her where she had been all day, and she told me she had been looking for an apartment. She didn't want to be here anymore.

I was angry. Not only did she take off all day without telling me where she was going, but there was no food in the house. Didn't she know I depended on her? I couldn't drive, and I needed her to get dinner for the kids and me.

Melanie just walked around ignoring me. She told me I could call my mother; that I had other options.

She kept walking away to avoid me. I was in a lot of pain

by this time. I had a tremendous headache and I couldn't take it anymore. It wasn't right being left alone in this condition with the full responsibility of the kids. I didn't know what to do anymore, and she wouldn't listen to me.

I sat down in my wheelchair, and Melanie walked off downstairs. I felt an energizing surge of rage that lifted me out of my wheelchair. I got up, walked downstairs and backed her into a corner. I wasn't myself at that point. When she saw the look in my eyes, she could tell she had pushed me too far.

I said, "You have this coming," and I raised my hand up. I was going to let her have it. Even in my condition I was mad enough that she knew she didn't stand a chance against me. I was at the brink of insanity. I had fire in my eyes.

As she had her hands up in front of her face, ready to protect herself, I heard the TV in the other room, and it brought my kids to mind. It was like a Big Hand reached in and pulled me back to reality. I realized if I did this I would probably be locked up and not see my kids for a long time. I looked at her and decided revenge wasn't worth it.

I walked off, and she ran from me. She told me she was going to leave with our daughter. I told her if she left Mallory with me she could leave, so she did. Soon after that, she showed up with the police on the front porch.

Melanie talked to the police for awhile, and I came out very calmly and sat on the porch. After the police talked to her, they came over and talked to me. I told them what was going on, and then they talked to the oldest boy for awhile. They came back and told me not to hit her, or I would go to jail. The police told Melanie this was between us, and they couldn't do anything. She got in the van and left. She slept in a motel that night.

CHAPTER 21

I was released from physical therapy and occupational therapy. I was walking more, and it was time for me to continue on my own. I had developed a pretty good relationship with my therapists. One of them was from Austria. All of my therapists were really neat people who enjoyed what they were doing. The therapists all cared about me. They were one of the most positive influences on my life, and I was going to miss that daily contact.

I realized I couldn't control what Melanie was going to do, so I called my mom and had her come and get me and the kids. When I told my mom how bad things were, we stayed with her for about a week.

Melanie called me to let me know she had found an apartment, and she wanted the kids to live with her. I wasn't in very good shape. I hadn't been eating right, and physically I was starting to go downhill. I agreed because I knew she loved the kids. We decided I would have them every other weekend.

I loved my kids and I missed them, but I knew I had take

better care of myself. I stayed at my mom's, so when I had the kids my mom could help me deal with their needs. Melanie said it was over, but I still figured if I just gave her time, she would come around and see that we could be a family again because I was changing. Maybe Melanie would realize that we both had problems and needed each other.

Time went on, and it was my weekend to have the kids. I had just gotten my kids, and we were eating dinner at my mom's house when the phone rang. It was my dad. When I got on the phone, he sounded pretty upset. I asked him what was wrong and he told me Grandpa was dying.

Earlier the doctors had thought it was pneumonia, but he had gone into the hospital where they found out it was terminal lung cancer. He had only a few weeks to live. I couldn't believe it. Things had just calmed down.

Every time things calm down, I get nervous. I keep waiting for the other shoe to drop. That's what happened: The other shoe had dropped. He was the only grandpa I had ever known on that side of the family. I couldn't believe this was happening.

When I got off the phone, my mom asked me what was wrong and I explained that my grandpa was dying, and I wanted to go to the coast and see him. I called Melanie and told her I needed to bring the kids back. She said she wasn't up to it and asked if I had any other options. I really had to press her as I felt I needed to leave right away.

Finally she agreed to take the kids. I went to her apartment to drop them off and she wasn't there. I kept trying to call from my brother's house until midnight, but she was out.

In the morning I went over with the kids and asked where she had been. She told me she had left before I got there the night before, because she couldn't handle having the kids. She said I needed to take them when it was my turn no matter what, because she couldn't handle things very well. She had been sitting in her car the night before, contemplating suicide. That really scared me. I could imagine being divorced, but I couldn't handle not seeing her forever.

I was so worried about seeing my grandpa, I didn't know what to do. Melanie told me again to find other options. Having no other choice, I told her, "Okay, my mother will have to watch them." My mother had plans for the weekend, but she canceled them. After I took my kids back over to my mother's house, I went with my brother down to the coast to see my grandpa.

CHAPTER 22

When my brother, Thom, and I finally arrived, Grandpa was sitting at the kitchen table looking out the window. Grandma and Grandpa Soderlund's house at the coast overlooks the ocean.

When I walked in, the first thing I noticed was that he had an oxygen tank running. I was shocked by how much weight he had lost. He used to be a big man, six feet seven inches and 275 pounds. He looked like he had lost about 100 pounds. He was so skinny he didn't look like himself anymore.

My brother and I went in, sat down and began to gracefully dance around the issue of dying. Grandpa was from the old school. He had served in the Korean War and had had a hard life. Grandpa was raised in Minnesota; the youngest son of seven children. His parents were Swedish immigrant farmers. His father had been in his sixties when Grandpa had been born. They were dirt poor; unable to afford any livestock or even a tractor. So Grandpa being the biggest and youngest of the children was forced by his father to pull a plow. Grandpa doesn't remember being told " I love you " or ever getting a hug.

One summer, after he was done with his chores, he sold firecrackers so he could earn enough money to buy a bicycle. After working and saving all summer he bought one and proudly brought it home. His father took it from him, sold it and kept the money.

When he was seventeen he lied about his age to join the army during the Korean War. Because he was so large and strong he was assigned to carry the machine gun which placed him on the front lines; he was the first one to be shot at by the enemy. Not long after he was fighting in Korea he was separated form his platoon and was lost in the Korean wilderness for three days. He never talked much to anyone about his war experiences. All he would say was "I know what its like to be hungry."

After his rescue, he was put back on the front lines. His best friend was always next to him when they were fighting. During one of the battles he saw him get blown up by a hand grenade. This same grenade also sprayed him with shrapnel. He was sent home. Every once in a while he would still dig out a piece of shrapnel from his skin.

My brother and I sat there with him swapping stories. Sometimes he would get serious and tell us, "Well, I guess I'm going to close this chapter of my life. I'm going to die, and there isn't much I can do about it."

I didn't know what to say so I was glad he was being blunt about it. He looked at me and said, "You know the score. This isn't much different from what you went through, except I don't have much hope of living."

He and I had a lot in common. We both had a history of dealing with our pain in the same way. We both had even spent some time in Damacsh, the state mental hospital, for fighting with the cops while in a drunken rage. When I was nineteen I had smashed my truck into a tree when I was drunk. I got out and started smashing the windows of my truck with my fists. When half a dozen police showed up, I foolishly turned on them trying to fight my way out. They were unable to control me even with their clubs. They threw me in a cruiser and drove me straight to the mental hospital where I could be restrained. I was there for a week. I remember my grandpa telling me he was going to come and bust me out. He had there himself for the exact same thing twenty years earlier.

We visited through the day. My dad was there, and he told us not to spend the night, because Grandma was so upset. We agreed to head back that night.

While we were driving home I asked God why was He letting this happen now. I had hoped to get closer to my grandpa now that I had the time. He was someone I could respect; we always seemed to connect, and now he was going to die. I guess things don't always work out the way we want them to.

I got back to Portland late that night. The next day I called Grandma to see how things were going. The news wasn't good. She said he was getting worse faster than the doctors had thought.

On Sunday night I got the kids ready to go back to Melanie's. When I took them to the apartment, she asked me how my grandpa was. I said, "Well, he's dying." That was all there was to it. I couldn't explain how I was feeling. I had mixed emotions and I didn't know how to describe them.

That week I stopped by to see the kids. As I was leaving, Melanie threw her arms around me and started crying. She said that she just needed some time to sort things out. She had done this a couple of times before. This would give me a bit of hope. I wondered if she was having second thoughts.

I was seeing my counselor, who encouraged me to detach from her. He warned me not to take what she said too seriously. She needed to deal with the issue of divorce herself and not drag me into it. If she was going to divorce me, it had to be her decision. I mustn't put pressure on her one way or the other. If she wanted a divorce, she was going to have to file herself.

The next time I saw my wife, she acted cold again, and I felt angry for letting myself hope. She behaved so inconsistently. She would say one thing and act another way. I was confused.

My grandpa progressively got worse. A week after I had last seen him, he asked me to come see him again. I went down to the coast by myself. He could still sit at the table and talk. Whenever Grandma and my step-mom left to take a break, I think he was relieved. Besides, he wanted to talk to me alone. We talked about life. My grandpa had been married more than once. He understood what I was going through.

He gave me a gold coin he had kept for a long time. It was a Canadian coin. He said as long as I had it, I would never be broke; because if the economy ever went bad, gold would always be worth something. He wanted me to have something to remember him by. I was touched. Even though we hadn't spent a lot of time together through the years; we realized now a special bond existed between us and we were a lot alike in many ways.

We talked through the day about things. We talked about Korea and all the crazy things he did when he was young. We talked about motorcycles, because I used to ride motorcycles. For the past twenty-five years he and my grandma had ridden Goldwing Hondas all over the United States. He told me the hardest thing for my grandma to give up was sitting behind him riding down the highways. They had just fulfilled their dream and bought a 1994 candy-apple red Goldwing. They hadn't been able to spend much time on it, and now it was sitting in the garage.

Before I went home back home, I told my grandma that I would come down again and help if she needed me to. My grandpa had the option of dying in the hospital, but he wanted to die at home.

The doctors told my grandma what it would be like; that he would slowly drown. They could give him enough morphine and other pills so that he wouldn't be in pain, but it wouldn't be a pretty sight. Deep down, I didn't want to witness this, but I knew it was important to my grandpa and grandma that they knew I could be there if they wanted me.

I didn't think they would take me up on it but my grandma said, "I may need you. Your grandpa doesn't want to have very many people around him. You're probably one of the few people he would want to be here and see him like this. I'm sure it will be okay. I will talk to him about it because I am going to need help."

CHAPTER 23

I went home to my mom's. The rest of the week I walked around in a daze. I tried to do exercises and eat better. Once in awhile I talked to my wife. I had the feeling things weren't going very well. All she did was complain about her problems.

She was changing. When I went over to her apartment, it was a mess and the kids' behavior was deteriorating. They were having a lot trouble with anger and whined all the time. They were fighting with each other and once and a while hit their mother. The oldest was withdrawing.

Despite my concern, when my grandma called and asked me to come and stay with her until my grandpa died, I put my life on hold and went.

I walked into my grandparents' house and my grandpa was sitting in his usual place at the kitchen table looking out over the Pacific Ocean. He had a wonderful view of Haystack Rock. I could tell by the way Grandpa was leaning on his arm that he didn't have much strength left. We started talking small talk; nothing too threatening. Grandma left us alone, and for a while we sat in silence.

My grandpa began to talk. He told me about the time years ago when he was with his first wife. He had come home early from a business trip and found her in bed with his best friend. He told me he beat the guy so bad that he almost died and it was all he could do to keep from killing her. Shortly after that they were divorced and he was awarded custody of his children. After he had them for awhile he agreed to sign papers sharing custody. It was hard taking care his kids alone without any help from his family. His ex-wife took them and moved to Canada without his permission. She refused to let him see his children. After several years of fighting with the Canadian authorities he was granted visitation. When he finally got to see them he discovered their mother had turned them against him by telling them lies. They thought he was a monster. He never saw them again while they were growing up.

My grandpa then told me about his second wife. She was a good woman, but he sabotaged that marriage. He was bitter, drank a lot and cheated on her. Finally she told him she couldn't take any more. One day he came home, and the house was empty. I could see the pain and regret on his face.

He looked me straight in the eye and said that the

bitterness and anger he had carried in his heart he felt had destroyed his life and was putting him an early grave at sixty-two years old. He said he had never learned how to forgive anyone.

We took a break from our heavy conversation and talked about the new motorcycles that were out on the market. We cracked a few jokes and talked about the basketball game and the weather.

Everyday he was growing weaker. On the day before Thanksgiving, the hospital bed arrived. He sat there and looked at it like it was a coffin. We didn't say it, but we both knew that once he got into that bed he would never get out of it alive. He was in no hurry to go over and try it out.

Grandpa commented that it looked comfortable. I told him, "They adjust to all kind of positions. I know. I was in one for quite a while."

He sat there for a long time just staring at the table. All of a sudden my grandpa looked up at the ceiling, then at the floor and then, as if he had been given a military command, he straightened up and said, "Well, I guess I better get in that bed."

As I got ready to go to bed that night, instead of the usual handshake, I hugged him. I said, "I love you, Grandpa. Hang in there, and I'll see you in the morning."

He raised his head up and gave me the biggest smile I had

ever seen him give. I knew it meant a lot to him.

It took facing death to bring the barriers down. He came to see me when I was in the hospital and grabbed my toe. That time and this were the only times we were able to express our feelings for each other.

Thanksgiving morning came. My grandma had been up with him all night. No one felt like baking a turkey, so we had meatloaf instead. We got a plate ready for Grandpa, but instead he called me to come and get him. I started to protest that he should save his strength, but instead I said nothing. By golly, if he wanted to eat Thanksgiving dinner at the table, he was going to. Even if it was meatloaf.

His arms were so weak he almost fell into his food, but he made it through dinner, and I helped him back to bed.

By Saturday it really wasn't him anymore. He only was conscious for a few minutes at a time, and his mind was clouded. None of us could stand to see him suffer anymore.

I got to the place where I contemplated putting the pillow over his face. My beliefs kicked in. I knew that no matter how much I wanted it to end, I could not take things in my own hands. I prayed and asked God to take him, but I did know it was not my decision to make.

My purpose right then was to make Grandpa as comfortable as possible. I wanted to leave and not have to see him die but I knew I had a job to do and when I accepted that it made it easier for me. I wanted to be there for him until the end, regardless of how I felt. He had been there for me when I was in ICU in really bad shape.

My grandma got so tired that she was seeing double and couldn't concentrate anymore. I took a short nap and then let my grandma go to bed. I sat up the rest of the night listening to his every breath. I kept wondering if each one was going to be his last. Several times I thought, *This is it, this is the last one*; then he would start breathing again.

I talked to him about all the places he had been. I talked to him about motorcycles even though I didn't know if he heard me or not. My grandma woke up Sunday morning, and we took turns sitting with him. She held his hand and told him, "It's okay honey, just let go. It's time to go."

Finally, the last breath came. I had never actually seen anyone die before. It wasn't so terrifying, I was happy for him. I was sad for me. The tears began running down my face. I didn't cry for long though. I got up and looked at him, but it wasn't him anymore.

I was reminded of the time when I was in ICU and was facing death. The only thing that mattered at that point was that I knew where I was going after I died. I thought about how my mom had told me when she had known Grandpa, he had shared with her how at one point in his life he had accepted the Lord as his savior before so many things had gone wrong for him. He was gone, but I had peace he was with the Lord now. I went into the kitchen, sat in Grandpa's chair at the table and looked out over the ocean.

Grandma called the funeral home. I went down to the coffee shop and had a cup of coffee and a Danish. I didn't know what else to do. The funeral director came and was very professional. The rest of the day my grandma, my step-mom and I wandered around. I think that we were all relieved it was over.

After a couple days I knew it was time to head home. I was supposed to have had my children for Thanksgiving, but I had canceled. It was time to get back to my life.

As I drove back to Portland I thought about all the things Grandpa and I had talked about. I could see I had a lot of anger and bitterness in my heart that I didn't know how to deal with. I knew Grandpa had been trying to tell me not to make the same mistakes he had. I wanted to teach my children to be loving and forgiving people but how in the world was I going to teach them when I didn't know how myself? As I drove, I felt like he was there with me telling me to live different. I didn't really understand how I was going to change but with God's help, I was going to find a way; for me, for my children and for Grandpa Joe.

CHAPTER 24

When I got home I called my wife. She asked me to take the kids for a week. I was happy to, because I missed them. When they came over, it was hard because their behavior had gotten to where they whined and cried most of the time. They were very upset, confused children.

I knew that they weren't getting what they needed and I could see that the separation was having terrible effects on them. Something needed to be done for them but I just didn't know what to do. I had grown up in a broken home and I could understand what they were going through. I didn't want them to have to face life with the kind of problems that come from having divorced parents.

I had tried hard at our marriage but we had established an unhealthy relationship. I always blamed myself for all our problems. When the stress or pressure got too much for me, I would get frustrated and lose my temper; then I would feel guilty and do whatever I could to try and fix things. But now, I could see that we both had problems. I felt like that with

God's help there could be hope for us.

My wife kept insisting that I had to let her go. She told me she was close to suicide, because she couldn't handle the pressure I was putting on her.

I didn't understand why she couldn't see what was so obvious to me and why she was so unwilling to try and save our marriage. Couldn't she see what was happening to our children?

CHAPTER 25

My third surgery was coming up. The doctors were going to hook up the nerves to the paralyzed side of my face. I wasn't looking forward to another surgery. The thought of surgery provoked strong emotions. I was still gun shy.

I saw Dr. Canepa the day before surgery and he explained the risks; all of which I had heard before. The next day was December 5th, the day of my surgery, and it was only my mom and me this time. I didn't have my wife and children or all my relatives waiting for me. Compared to my last surgeries this would be a walk in the park. There is always risk when you have surgery, but it was minimal this time.

I recognized the person who came to wheel me down for surgery. I had spent so much time in this hospital, it seemed like I knew everyone there. I was in the same pre-op room for the third time. I wondered if that was a good sign, or a bad sign. I had a different anesthesiologist, but I was comfortable with him. I was checked in, and once again rolled through the double doors.

The operating room was different. It was a smaller, brighter room, and the table wasn't stainless steel but a soft, padded table with lots of blankets. It made it easy to adjust. I jumped off the gurney and climbed on the table. The nurses were standing around. It got to be noon, and Dr. Canepa was late.

I started talking to the nurses and told one of them, "Make sure they sew me up this time." She looked at me puzzled and asked me what I meant. I told them how at my last surgery the doctor had forgotten to sew up the incision behind my right knee.

They all said, "What!"

I explained and just as they all started laughing, Dr. Canepa walked in. He walked over to me and asked "What's so funny?"

The nurses wouldn't say anything; the cowards.

I decided to tell him. "I was just telling the nurses to make sure you sewed me up this time."

He grinned, then told me it was his partner who had overlooked it.

As the anesthesiologist put me out, my last thought was, *Gee, maybe it wasn't a good idea to get Dr. Canepa riled up just before he does my surgery.*

When I woke up in the post-op room, the pain was intense. My face was throbbing. Dr. Canepa gave me something in my IV, and I felt a warm feeling as I went out again. When I woke up the next time, I was on my way to my room on the eighth floor.

Coming back in this hospital room was like returning to a war zone after the battle was over. It was much calmer this time. I was able to think clearly.

I sat and stared out the window, remembering. I realized I was changing. I had more peace. I could deal with life. I was better at processing my emotions. I was beginning to find myself.

I was grateful for time to think things over. Before I had my first surgery, I had lost my sense of self in all my busyness. My illness had helped me discover the kind of man I was.

At midnight as the anesthetic began to wear off, I discovered I was tremendously hungry. I knew they had a good menu at this hospital. However, when I was here the first time I couldn't eat solid food the entire time. I asked for a menu and ordered a fresh fruit platter and manicotti.

When the food came I couldn't believe it. I had never seen anything like it in a hospital before. The fruit platter was half of a decoratively carved cantaloupe with piles of grapes, strawberries, honeydew melon, and pineapple. It was huge. The manicotti was fresh and not a microwave special. It was a feast! It was like dining at the Hilton.

At the end of my feast, I leaned back with satisfaction. It was a wonderful meal. This pleasure was short-lived. The pain came back, and it was like being pounced on by a lion. The pain was intense and throbbing.

After trying every position to stop hurting, I ended up sitting on the edge of the bed staring at the floor. So much for trying to be macho. I called for some pain medication. I couldn't believe how quickly the pain disappeared. I could see how pain pills could be addictive. On Demerol, I loved everybody.

I had trouble, but I did sleep some. To say the least, I was not happy to have the nurse wake me up at seven the next morning. I was glad to have breakfast, but shortly after that the lion pounced again. The pain was less than after my brain surgery, but now I was more alert. All I could do was sit on the side of my bed and stare at the floor.

Dr. Canepa came in about 8:30 A. M. and asked me if I wanted to go home. He told me he would keep me as long as I wanted to stay, because I had been through so much.

The pain became more and more uncontrollable. Another medication was added, but it didn't seem to help. One nurse believed it was because one of my old scars had been reopened. Many different medications were tried during the day to bring my pain back to a level I could stand. That night I couldn't get beyond the pain to fall asleep.

One of the things I learned from all the pain I had been through the past year was that sometimes I just have to endure it. Pain is the first step on the avenue of healing. Facing my pain instead of avoiding it helped me practice concentrating on the process of moving through the pain and fighting the battles in my mind.

While I was in the hospital, Melanie brought the kids to see me. She came in and rushed over to my bed, acting very concerned. She asked me how I was doing and if I was in pain. I told her the surgery went well, but, yes, I was in pain.

After five minutes, without me asking her, she started talking about how stressed out she was, how terrible her finances were, and how she couldn't handle the kids. I could see that her concern for me was short lived. There was one thing I felt sure about right then: she really did not care about me that much.

After enduring her complaints for a few minutes, I told her I really was in a lot of pain and not up to visiting. She became sober faced and left. It may seem strange, but I felt very safe there in the hospital. It was nice to have time to reflect and not be responsible for everything and have people take care of me.

After three days Dr. Canepa came in and wanted to release me. The problem was that I was living on Demerol every hour to control the pain. I was given a different pain medication. My mom came to get me, and I took one last shot of Demerol. I had to sit in the wheelchair, because the medication made it hard to walk.

Finally, my doctor found an extra strength prescription that seemed to work, but that evening I was watching television when I started drifting. It felt similar to the time I spent in ICU. I lay down, feeling as if I was going to float away. It scared me, because I was afraid I was having neurological problems again.

My mother called Dr. Roher who reassured me by saying that having another surgery so soon could bring a relapse of the symptoms. He prescribed a medicine to deal with the feeling of drifting, which helped some. It occurred to me that whatever the symptoms, the medical profession would find a pill for it.

Gradually over the next few days, the pain subsided. I was over the hurdle again. Now all I had do was wait a few months to see if my face would show any signs of moving. After that it could take two to five years before I would know how much movement I would regain. I have never been a patient person. How was I ever gong to handle waiting so long?

CHAPTER 26

Christmas time came. Every time I went to my wife's apartment to pick up my children, it looked like a pigsty. The kids always looked tired.

While I still didn't believe I was capable of full time parenting, I could see the lack of stability in their lives. In spite of the fact I was still recovering, I was concerned and considered the possibility of getting custody. At this point I still believed the reason Melanie was a mess was because I had let her down.

Christmas lights were up, and it started to feel like Christmas. I remembered when I was a child I would get up in the middle of the night and turn on the tree lights and lie there under the tree and enjoy feeling warm and safe. Despite all the chaos of growing up and the rough times, at Christmas we always felt like a family.

My mind was clearing and my strength was coming back. I had always assumed I needed to give my wife custody of the kids. I felt I wasn't capable of raising them, but I could see she wasn't doing a good job. I was going to counseling on a regular basis, and I began to gain confidence in my ability to raise the kids myself. I thought to myself, *Maybe the reason God has restored me is so I can raise my children.*

Christmas week I was supposed to have the kids all week. When I picked them up, Melanie told me she was going into the psychiatric ward for observation because of her suicidal thoughts. I asked her to speak to her doctors because she still had custody of the kids and I wanted to know if she was able to take care of them, however, she did not want me to be involved at all.

After I had the kids for three days, they settled down. We got a tree. It was late in the season, but as we prepared for Christmas and did a little shopping, they seemed to lose the feeling that the whole world was coming to an end. It was Christmas time, and everything would be okay for awhile.

On Christmas Eve Melanie called and asked me to bring the kids to her mother's house. She was out of the hospital on a pass. I agreed. When I got there she kept hugging me, being sweet and giving signals that she wanted to be with me. She flirted as the night went on. I don't think she realized how she was building up my hopes, and it sure played havoc on my emotions.

When I got ready to leave, she told me she still loved me. That did it. I still wanted to be reconciled and this was just the icing on the cake.

On Christmas Day Melanie asked me to bring the kids up to the ward to see her. The patient's families were invited to visit, and they had food set out so families could eat together. I didn't want to blow my chances, since she had been so warm the night before, so I changed my plans, got the kids all dressed up, and went to see her. She was extremely cold to me. I went home very depressed.

The next day I went to see her by myself. We sat in the lounge, and after some small talk I asked her if she had reconsidered. Her whole body language and reaction showed how shocked she was. She became very upset and told me emphatically that she had never given me any indication that she had changed her mind. She was aghast at the whole idea. I had to learn to leave her alone and let her go.

I had nothing more to say. How do you reply to someone who tells you that what happened didn't happen? I didn't see what I saw, feel what I felt, or hear what I heard.

My counselor pointed out to me I wasn't just receiving mixed signals; she was sending mixed signals. I think Melanie really didn't want to be married to me, but she didn't want to let me out of her control either.

I had to come to terms with the fact that my wife had decided not to stay married to me. I know now that you can't control people, only yourself. I still wanted to work on our marriage, but I had to accept her choice.

Now my wife, who only a few months earlier had left me to find herself and feel fulfilled, was in the psychiatric ward because she was suicidal. Logically, this didn't fit together. Usually if you are in a bad relationship and you get away from it, you start getting better. She was getting worse. It made me wonder if there was more going on than I had been aware of.

I had always felt that I was the one who could fix Melanie; but no matter how much I tried to change, it didn't change things for her. This was a clue that helped me see the truth that I wasn't the cause of all her problems, as I believed.

When Melanie got out of the hospital, she had planned to take the kids again. She said they had adjusted her medicine and she felt fine. I was concerned, but there wasn't much I could do.

At the last minute, she changed her mind and asked me to keep the kids another night. It was New Year's Eve, and I had made plans to spend time with my grandmother. She didn't want to spend New Year's Eve alone so soon after Grandpa's death.

I told Melanie that I didn't appreciate the last minute change and how important this was to my grandmother. She called me a jerk and insisted that I needed to support her emotionally. I wondered how I could be a support to her unless I was her husband. I called my grandmother and canceled.

CHAPTER 27

I cried out to the Lord and asked Him why I was still getting hurt. One night as I was driving home, the emotions I had managed to keep from erupting suddenly exploded. I yelled and told God I couldn't take any more.

When I got home I stood in the basement and begged God to fix my marriage and take away the pain. But somehow I knew this was the wrong prayer. I felt God was telling me to pray that His will be done. I didn't want to pray for God's will for my marriage. It was too hard. I just didn't want to let go. I was reminded of when I was in the hospital and feeling like there was no hope and I had asked God to die. Here I was dealing with something that was too big for me again. I knew God needed to take control of this situation. Finally, I bowed my and head and prayed, *Not my will, Lord, but your will be done.*

When I went to bed that night, I fell asleep crying. I was scared, but I also felt relieved.

When I talked to Melanie afterward, I sensed a difference in myself. Usually, when we had disagreements I would either attack or retreat. Now, I decided what was right and stood up for myself. I didn't get nearly as angry. I wouldn't defend myself. I would just stick to the truth.

I had a couple weeks with no obligations, so I went to see my grandmother.

We talked about my grandpa's death. My grandma cried a lot, and I was there to comfort her. We also spent time on the beach.

It felt nice to be at peace. I wondered what bombshell would drop next.

CHAPTER 28

I was due to have the kids on Friday. Melanie called on Wednesday and asked me to take them early. I agreed, so she came over and quickly unloaded their things. The kids seemed very upset. She hugged the kids and left quickly.

Richard was whimpering and pulled away from me. He was sick. Mallory kept kicking and screaming and yelling for her mom. Finally, I got Mallory calmed down.

Bryan, my stepson, made a beeline for the television. It was as if something horrible had happened.

By this time, Richard was under my mother's bed. When I finally got Mallory to talk, the first thing she said was, "I've been keeping a secret from you, Daddy."

They knew that we didn't keep secrets in our family. Mallory told me she couldn't tell me, that if she told me the secret, I would get very upset and hurt Mommy or hurt them. It was upsetting to see my kid's feeling this much turmoil. Mallory told me that Mommy had a friend.

I asked if it was a new friend, and she said no, it was Mark. I said, "You mean, Mom's old boss named Mark?"

She said, "Yeah. He spends the night sometimes, and other times Mommy and I go to his house and we spend the night there. Mommy, told me I couldn't tell you, because you would be angry."

Richard and Bryan also told me that the secret was about Mark spending the night, and they were told not to tell me. I was stunned.

I sat down and put the pieces together. I recalled how easily Melanie got the job when I first got out of the hospital; and then was quickly promoted. It had to have been because of Mark. No wonder he treated me so funny at the company picnic last summer. I suspected something was wrong when she would stay out all night after work, but I had buried my suspicions. Now I knew it was all true. I felt like I had been body slammed by a professional wrestler.

I started crying, even though I didn't want to cry in front of my kids. My daughter tried to comfort me. After several minutes, the anger began to well up in me. I wanted to hurt both Melanie and Mark. I had visions of choking him with my bare hands, or running him over with my car. I couldn't deal with it. I called my mom and asked her to come home and told her why.

I couldn't handle the onslaught of intense rage and shame

I was feeling. I called my doctor, and she contacted my counselor. They wanted me go to the hospital so I could work through what was happening to me. I agreed to go because I wanted to be somewhere safe where I couldn't do anything I would regret.

The psychologist on duty explained to me that when a person has been through as much as I had in a short period of time, there comes a moment when you can't handle any more emotionally. It is like lifting weights. Eventually you get too weary. The weight is more than you can carry, and you have to set it down for awhile.

It was a wise thing for me to spend some time away in the hospital. The psychologist asked me if I felt like I might get violent, so they could take precautions. I explained that I was only angry with my wife and her boyfriend, because she had started going out on me during the lowest time of my life. They were relieved that I understood the problem.

The staff psychologist prescribed an antidepressant sleeping pill for me. I still couldn't fall asleep until midnight.

I woke up the next day and felt hungover. I was very depressed. The nurses offered to help me, if I needed it. I spent most of the day wandering around the ward, sometimes visiting with other patients.

I went to a group and was very quiet at first, because I was used to talking to a counselor, one-on one. The psychologist came by and talked to me alone later that evening. He told me I was not insane, and I was right to ask for help. The doctor told me that even he was capable of needing professional help.

The doctor and I agreed that I would have to confront my wife about her unfaithfulness, but in a non-threatening way. We did some role playing. He played the role of my wife and came up with excuses and denials, while I practiced confronting her. This helped me a lot.

I was also helped with the emotional pain I was feeling. I had to learn to deal with the reality that she could make choices over which I had no control that were painful to me. At the same time, I had to value myself. What had happened was a tragedy, but I could move on.

I faced the fact that I was incredibly angry, partly because I was in incredible pain. I wanted to lash out and hurt the people who hurt me. By the second day I was taking the doctors' advice and letting the hurt flow and the tears fall. I let it hurt and be painful. I didn't try to stop it.

When my brother, Thom, came to visit me, I was still crying. I don't think he had ever seen me this way before. He sat across from me and looked at me. He talked to me a little. He asked me questions, and I told him I never thought I could feel this much hurt. I told him I hoped he never had to go through this.

The Bible says that two become one flesh. I understood the truth of this because I felt torn apart. Even though we had had a rough marriage, and she turned out to be a different person than I thought she was, I still felt connected to her. I had a broken heart. Something had been torn away from me, and it was gone.

My brother sat there while I cried. Just like the pain I went through after all my surgeries, I knew I had to endure this. I had hope that if I experienced the pain of facing the truth, I would once again find healing in my life. I asked the Lord to help me and show me what to do so I could move on.

I stood at my fifth floor window and watched the rain. I saw two seagulls flying and felt like the Lord was speaking to me. I realized that no matter what was happening in the world, or what problems existed below them, the birds would still fly. I felt better. It was God's way of comforting and helping me realize I would get through this time, and the pain would be over some day. It gave me hope that some day I would fly again.

I began to realize then that I needed to get my children. I was important to them. I was their Dad. I needed to heal, so I could be there for them. I knew what I was going through was horrible, but they were also suffering and needed attention. Things were going to be hard for them.

CHAPTER 29

I got in my car and headed for my counselor's office. The closer I got, the sicker I felt. I remembered when my kids were born. I remembered our wedding and the good times we had together. Now it was destroyed. When I went to work in the mornings, I used to dream about raising our kids, then retiring, spending time traveling, and doing things together. None of this was going to happen.

I went into my counselor's waiting room. As I waited, I sat in the lobby and cried. I had never cried in front of total strangers before, but I couldn't help it. It felt like my whole life was coming to an end. The Lord was beginning to give me a vision of a new life; but to have this new life, I had to keep surrendering the old life.

With my counselor, Craig, I put in a conference call to my wife. She told me she was afraid to talk to me in person. During the conference call, I told Melanie what the kids had told me about Mark spending the night. She denied it.

She told me Mark was just a friend. They spent time

together; although something might develop later, they were just good friends. Mark was a person who was there for her, while she was going through a hard time. I didn't believe her, but there wasn't much I could say.

I stayed and talked to Craig for awhile about learning how to let go. I realized I had formed a strong habit of accepting what she said as true. Even though I knew the truth, the old records played, and I was tempted to listen to them. A part of me wanted to believe what she was saying was true. That maybe there was still a shred of hope we could put our marriage back together but I knew she was lying. I had to accept that and go on from there.

Reflecting on this, I think Melanie was also trying to protect Mark. When she had asked me if I was going retaliate, it was a giveaway that I had a reason to be upset and she had lied. I told her I wasn't going to do anything to Mark.

As I drove back to the hospital, I felt like I had gained some freedom; like a burden had been lifted from me. God had come and touched me. This gave me the courage to believe I could change and get out of my old habit patterns.

CHAPTER 30

When I got back to the hospital, the nurse who evaluated me said she could see a difference in me. In the morning Dr. Beamer talked to me and told me I was free to go home. He told that he believed I had dealt with my situation and learned a great deal. He thought I would be fine as I continued counseling.

I began to look forward to working through things with my counselor. It used to seem so overwhelming to me that I hated to even go to counseling. Now that I knew the truth, I was finished trying to please Melanie. I was free to hope, to let go of the past and go on with my life. I realized how true the Scripture was that I would know the truth and the truth would set me free. (John 8:32)

I had been spared for a purpose. God was at work to change me. With the Word of God and through counseling, I was going to be healthy. God was setting me free.

The kids stayed with me for extended periods of time. I never knew when I was going to have them. I wanted full custody but Melanie was opposed to the idea. It seemed like she wasn't handling the burden of caring for them very well. She was changing rapidly. Every time I saw her, she had a new hair style or different clothes or new makeup. I wondered if she was fighting me about the kids strictly because it was my idea.

I never mentioned Mark again. When I saw Melanie, I was calm. God was giving me peace. I realized when I had my kids, I was happy. I missed them when they weren't with me. I felt close to them.

One day Melanie called and told me to come get the kids and keep them. She told me she couldn't handle them any more. They didn't have food or heat in the house, and she was going to give me custody of my two kids, but not my stepson. I went over immediately. She was busy packing their clothes and told me she thought they would be better off with me.

I sat down and talked to her one last time about our marriage. She reaffirmed that it was over, so I agreed to talk to a lawyer. When I took the kids home with me, I thought the subject of where the kids would live was settled.

My kids told me that sometimes they had gone without eating. This made me feel bad because I had given her money for them and had bought them groceries regularly. It was hard for them to talk about things. They didn't want to betray their mom. She had told them in the past not to tell me things that happened at her house.

The next two weeks I got reacquainted with my children. It took a week for their behavior to settle down, and then I began to enjoy the responsibility of raising kids.

At the end of the third week, Melanie called and said she was ready for them to come home now. I asked her if she meant for the weekend.

"No", she said. "I have been doing a lot of thinking, and I want the children to come home now."

I reminded her that only three weeks ago, she told me she would give me the house and the kids, because she couldn't raise them by herself. She said that she didn't really mean that I would have them permanently, but just until she got back on her feet. I told her I couldn't just give them back until we sat down and talked about some things.

Melanie had a new job now so she was ready to take my kids; just like that. When I asked her about them not having enough to eat, she denied that it had happened. She informed me that the kids were just making it up. There had never been a problem. Everything was fine now.

I told Melanie that I hadn't changed my mind. The kids were going to live with me. She got very upset and hung up.

Thursday evening I was driving home from a class, and as I looked in my rearview mirror, I saw a sheriff's car behind me. He followed me the rest of the way home. When I pulled in my driveway, a deputy came up and asked if I was Richard Jones.

When I said yes, he served me with a restraining order, ordering me to stay away from my wife.

I went into the house, and my mother told me the deputies had already come and taken the children. Melanie had told the police I refused to return the children after visitation.

The deputy sat down and started talking to me about the work he had done in the past with people who were brain damaged. I was appalled. Here was an officer of the law talking to me as if I had brain damage. Who knows what she had told them?

I don't think I even heard very much of what he said, I was so shocked. There wasn't much that I could do. Melanie had pulled a fast one. Obviously, she had this officer buffaloed.

My mother said the deputy had told her when he came in the house what a nice lady Melanie was. I felt like someone had come in and robbed me.

My lawyer called the next morning to see what was happening. He went through the roof when I read him the terms of the petition that I had been served. I had never hit my wife; so she told the judge she had to have the kids, because I was brain damaged and unstable. She didn't tell him she had turned the kids over to me willingly.

My lawyer told me that this meant war.

The last thing I wanted was war over my children, and now I had to fight for them. I knew now I could not trust anything Melanie said to me. I was going to have to proceed the way that I knew I should. I began a custody case and took the kids to a psychologist.

Melanie didn't stick to the terms of the petition. Whenever she wanted me to care for the kids, she would leave them with me. One time I had them for a month. This fight wasn't about who had the children. This fight was about who would have control of the decisions.

The war within was the struggle with feelings of wanting revenge. God was helping me to relax and enjoy my kids' company. I was in the process of discovering who I was as a person and a father.

As I concentrated on moving ahead, I surrendered my desire to repay Melanie in any way whatsoever. I moved in the confidence that my children should be with me.

I got married when I was twenty-one, and I know now that I had never learned to be a single person or someone who could rely on their own source of happiness. I had gotten married with my own set of problems and taken on all of her problems, too. I just wasn't mature enough. Now God was helping me to accept my aloneness and face the problems in my life. I didn't know much about being a father but I was sure God would help me to grow up and teach me what I needed to know. Learning patience would gain me the freedom to wait for what He had for me.

CHAPTER 31

I planned a string of activities with the kids, including hiking and camping. I avoided going to the movies or the video arcades, because I could see they needed more peaceful interactions with me.

One of the activities was a hike up Multnomah Falls in the Columbia River Gorge. There is a paved trail up to a bridge and then you can hike to the top of this waterfall. It is a fairly easy hike. I piled the kids in my little red Volkswagen Rabbit.

We stopped to see my insurance agent on the way, and as the agent chatted with my kids, he told my stepson Bryon, who was nine, that he didn't think Bryon could walk all the way to the top of Multnomah Falls without stopping. Bryon never turns down a challenge. He told the agent he was going to do it.

When we got to the lodge at the bottom of the falls, I waited for the two smaller kids. Bryon was eager to get going, so he quickly disappeared from sight. It took the three of us about a half-hour to make the climb. At the top, the trail goes down a short way to a platform that overlooks the top of the falls. Just as we rounded the top of the mountain we met Bryon, who informed us he had made it all the way without stopping.

However, because there were no bathrooms on the trail, he had an embarrassing accident. We hurried back to the car and headed for Portland thirty-five miles away. The odor got stronger and stronger. Bryon began howling with laughter, because we were all suffering. The others had the most quiet and peaceful trip ever, because they were busy holding their noses.

My little red Rabbit transformed into a race car as I drove speedily through fairly heavy traffic. My performance was flawless as I wove in and out of traffic in a marvelously efficient manner, especially considering I had my head hanging out the window. As we pulled into the driveway, the car was immediately vacated.

This unfortunate incident helped us pull away from our problems for awhile and let us just be people again. It was a fun month together.

We went camping where a squirrel invaded our campsite. This squirrel was so smart, he figured out how to undo the clasp on our food basket and eat our Hershey bars. I moved everything into the tent and we went for a walk in the woods.

When we came back we could see him in our tent. When he heard us coming, he tried to get out in a hurry. He had managed to unzip the tent and had eaten all our potato chips this time. He was the fattest little squirrel I had ever seen.

After a month of swimming, hiking and water fights, reality set in. The kids had to go back to their mother's. I was sad to see them go. I wished I could have them permanently. It was hard having someone else tell me when I could see my kids.

My lawyer told me things took time in divorce cases, so I went to see my dad so I could do some fishing and get my mind off of things for awhile. But it was hard to enjoy myself. I kept thinking about how I had just found out Mark had moved in with Melanie. It felt like my home had been invaded. This man had taken advantage of my weakness, and I didn't want my children around him.

I had doubts when Melanie had told me nothing was going on with Mark. I even doubted my children when she told me they were lying, but now there was no refuting their relationship. I had been told that what I saw and what I felt was not valid. Now my children were being told that what they had saw happening at their mother's house was not real, and they were just mistaken. It helped sever my feelings for her.

CHAPTER 32

One morning I woke up, and that feeling of wishing she was there was gone. The only feelings that seem to be left were betrayal, abandonment and a lot of anger towards her.

The night before when I was sleeping I awoke suddenly in a cold sweat. I don't remember the dream I was having but I know it was God that woke me because the memory of a dream that I had had when I was in ICU was vividly in my mind and I knew God was showing me what it meant. It was the one where I was in hell in a stone courtyard and there were the demons that looked like they were made of clay with the smallest one sitting on a throne and all the others obeying him out of fear. God told me that the small demon on the throne represented lust and that he was small because he was hidden. All of the other demons represented anger, envy, alcoholism, hate, fear and many others. They helped to hide him which gave him his power. He was the one who opened the door for all the others. The manifestation of this demon and his cohorts had plagued many generations in my family. I could see they had been there in my life too and had caused me a great deal of pain.

As I read the Bible to find more clarity I understood what could happen to people when these demons are not dealt with. I was also reading about forgiveness. The Bible says that when you do not forgive you will not be forgiven. When I was growing up I felt like bad things were always done to me and that others needed to ask me for my forgiveness. And now, after all that Melanie had done to me I felt that way even more so.

I wondered how I was going to be able to understand God's concept of forgiveness and I wondered how the meaning of my dream fit into all of this. Somehow I knew the dream and its meaning tied into the issue of forgiveness but I just couldn't put it all together.

CHAPTER 33

I went to see Dr. Canepa, my face surgeon. He was disappointed with the progress in my face. He discussed using part of the nerve to my tongue, but this would severely affect my speech. My speech was already affected somewhat, but it was still pretty good.

I didn't want to face another surgery. I was very disappointed. Depression came over me like a wave. I felt very helpless and upset. I had never accepted that half of my face would be paralyzed. I had thought that after a short period of time my face would go back to where it was before my brain surgery.

As I walked out the hospital door to my car, the depression built. I started the car, but I just sat there. I started screaming. I had gone through two surgeries for my face, and I didn't want the pain to be for nothing.

As I continued to yell, the yelling turned into crying. I looked in the mirror, and I could see the lifelessness on one side of my face. It was like a desert, barren. I didn't want to go through life with my face this way.

Finally I stopped crying and backed my car out. As I drove home, I realized there was nothing I could do. Either my surgery would eventually bring the nerves back in my face, or it wouldn't. This situation was another challenge for me not to let bitterness set in.

Once again, I was going to have to let go. The truth was the surgery might never work, and if I let bitterness grow the worse it would get. It was like a weed that twisted and tangled my emotions, and if I didn't deal with it, the bitterness would grow until it took over the whole garden.

Once again I prayed that the Lord's will would be done. I asked Him to help me so that whatever the outcome, God would help me accept it.

I called one of the neurosurgeons who had operated on me and talked to him about my face. He told me that this was a fairly rare surgery. No one really knew how long it would take for the nerves to recover. He said it could take up to a year to start seeing results.

It helped to know that this doctor had a different opinion, but once you have been afraid, it is hard to set it aside. I filed this information in my brain, but I still decided I would stick to my original plan of letting this go.

My face was important as a way to express my feelings;

it's where others read me. I noticed that people reacted differently to me since my face was paralyzed. Several times I had cracked a joke and had people stare at me for a minute, until they realized it was a joke, and then they would laugh. We depend on facial expressions as part of language and communication.

I realized I was going to have to communicate more verbally my feelings and expressions. This was frustrating for me. It was one more thing to deal with and to learn. I was looking forward to moving on, and I was having to relearn some of the basic things in communicating.

There is a lot of emphasis on looks in our society. It would be good for me to have to learn that outward attractiveness is only skin deep. It seemed it would be healthier to learn what a person is like on the inside and not go by the first thing I see. Even though losing my looks was hard, I knew I would look at others differently now.

CHAPTER 34

I felt fortunate to have my faith even though finding faith wasn't an easy road for me. It grew out of a series of choices to trust in God.

It started in the hospital when I couldn't move and I surrendered to God. I realized I couldn't control my situation, and came to the point where I wanted to die. I had to have the faith to tell God I couldn't change things. Out of my desperation and neediness I cried to God and I received the answer that I would walk. My recovery began at that point.

Now it was over a year later and I had given up my marriage, my face, my home and my vocation. It was like I had lost my identity and who I was. I needed faith and that faith didn't come from me. God gave it to me as I cried out to Him. I could see that even the process was orchestrated by the Lord.

Ideally, I should turn to God first, but even when I turned to Him as a last hope, He had enough grace and mercy to take control at that point. He didn't tell me since you didn't come to me first, I'm not going to help you. He was there for me.

Now that I had let go of my life, my face, my wife, I thought there wasn't much else to surrender to God. But there was one thing. Something I thought I would never have to let go of. But I couldn't let go of that. Not my children.

When I read the Bible or I would pray, I was starting to hear that I should let go of control of my children and let God finish His work. I understood that I was to lay down my weapons and let God take care of the custody issue. I had a custody lawsuit going. I was prepared for battle. I had documentation. I had primed my lawyer. I had the psychologist lined up, and I was ready to attack.

I was looking forward to my first strike. In this time of preparation for the battle for my kids, all my relatives and friends urged me to fight. It was a just and noble cause.

Even with all these confirmations from the world that I should fight, there was a voice deep inside of me urging me to let it go. I couldn't believe it! How could I not fight for my kids? This caused me a great deal of turmoil. I was depressed, I was unhappy. I was confused so again I left for my dad's at the coast to try and sort things out.

I had been there a couple of days so I called and talked to my kids. My daughter, Mallory, acted distant. My son, Richard, didn't even want to talk to me. Melanie came on the phone, and I told her I wanted to have the kids for a week as soon as I got back to Portland. She told me I could only see them on the two weekends a month that was allowed by the court.

She knew I was building a case against her, and she wasn't going to let me see them. I got furious and told her she couldn't just use the kids as pawns in a game. They wanted to be with me; they were my kids, and I didn't see how she could do this. She told me that was what I could expect from now on for trying to build a case against her.

I slammed the phone down after we had screamed at each other for a few minutes, and I went down to the beach and started running. Once again I began screaming. I screamed that I wanted her to pay. I wanted revenge. It was a good thing I was three hundred miles away. I felt like smashing things. I was so angry at her for withholding my children from me.

I ran along the beach for awhile, alternating between crying and yelling. When I was totally exhausted, I fell on my knees and told God I couldn't stand my kids being put in the middle. I was in absolute despair.

Just like the other times, this was when I heard God's voice the clearest. He simply told me, "Let it go. Don't fight it. Give in." I decided to drop the custody suit. I would give her the kids and see them as much as I could.

That was my plan.

I left my dad's and drove all night to get home. After I slept, the first thing I did was to call Melanie and tell her I had decided to drop the custody suit. I wasn't going to fight her for the kids.

That's when she told me that she had decided not to fight me. It was as if everything had been defused.

This was the first time in a year that I sensed peace between us and a decision based on what was best for the children. Melanie told me if I gave her the house and the computer and took my clothes and personal things, she would give me custody of the kids. She seemed very sincere and told me she wanted what was best for them. I was stunned.

I was amazed at what the Lord could do. Instead of having to play the game and walk the line to see my kids, the Lord had taken care of this situation. There would be no major battle with my kids caught in the middle. I had let go of my children, and God had kept them.

CHAPTER 35

Two weeks before Christmas 1996, things were peaceful at last. The kids were starting to settle down and get used to the idea of living with their dad. My ability to emotionally distance myself from Melanie and her life was becoming stronger. I had the feeling she wanted to talk to me about some things but I kept our conversations short and businesslike. My life was moving on in Christ. I felt that we didn't have any common ground between us except for the children.

Then late one night, I received a phone call. Melanie told me, "Now that we are divorced, I want to tell you all that went on." My first thought was, *Oh boy, here we go.* However, I felt that I should be patient and listen.

She started telling me that when I went to the coast to visit my dad after my surgery, my youngest brother seduced her into a night of passion by using alcohol and smooth talk.

When she told me this, it didn't seem to hurt that she had been unfaithful even more than what I had thought. I had already dealt with her unfaithfulness when I had found out about her and Mark. I can't say that I had forgiven her but I had emotionally detached from her and was unable to feel any more pain over what she had done.

However, while we were talking I could feel my blood running cold and a calm rage growing towards my brother for his betrayal. I told her, "I forgive you, but this has to be between you and God" I could tell she wanted more from me. All I wanted was to get off the phone. When I hung up I thought about when I was in the hospital on the psych ward, talking to my older brother Thom about how I didn't think I could feel much more emotional pain than my wife's infidelity. I was wrong; this was worse.

I thought, *I have every right to beat up my brother and disown him. It's time for some justified revenge No one would blame me. After all, when someone that close to you betrays you, they don't deserve any mercy. I'm not taking anymore!* My anger built as I calmly walked out of the house and drove to my brother's.

When I arrived at his house, I stormed to the door. He was not home. I went back to my car to wait.

Over the next hour I ignored God telling me to leave and talk to my counselor Craig, before confronting my brother. Instead I sat and thought about how I was going to pound him into the ground.

Finally, I got tired of waiting so I went home. I called my

older brother, hoping he would condone the acts of violence I was plotting against Steve.

Instead, Thom told me this was an attack from the enemy to split my relationship with my brother forever.

These words of truth angered me all the more. I argued that he deserved to be punished for what he had done. Thom tried to talk to me, but I wouldn't listen. When I hung up, my plans for revenge had not changed.

The next day I had an appointment with my counselor. After I finished telling him the story, he offered his opinion. My counselor asked me to consider the possibility that Melanie, by waiting so long to tell me was trying to alleviate her guilt and to shift the blame on my brother.

When I could see beyond my anger and sense of betrayal, I realized there were works of darkness here, and these people were victims of sin and adultery. When I saw this, my heart started to soften.

As I drove home, my mind journeyed through the years. My thoughts took me back to my wedding night. I remember making a vow to myself *If any other man touches my wife, I will show him no mercy.*

At that point, the rage rekindled. I decided despite what God had to say about mercy, I would keep my vow. I felt I had earned the right when I married her.

For the rest of the drive, I plotted against my brother.

Maybe a round house kick to the side of the head? Maybe a straight punch to the nose? If I could break his nose, he would be blind for a few seconds, plenty of time to inflict damage to him. By the time I arrived at his house I was ready. I had my plan worked out. I was going to beat him up like he deserved and then disown him.

My brother answered the door. He could tell right away something was wrong. As he led the way to his room, he kept looking back over his shoulder. Maybe he could feel my anger?

When we got to his room, he walked in, and I slammed the door. At that, he spun around and said, "What is it?" With my fist clenched in anger, I told him that I had talked to Melanie. As I talked, I could see the strength draining from his body. He looked like a flower wilting.

Finally he sat on his bed, hung his head low and started to cry. He said that he didn't even like her, but he had betrayed me, and he deserved to die. He was at my mercy.

Just as I was getting ready to carry out my plan, I heard that Voice again. The Lord said to me, *"It is finished."*

I stopped and said in my mind, *"I don't understand."*

The Lord told me that I needed to forgive my brother. I told Him *" I'm not able to forgive this and anyway, Steve doesn't deserve it."* Then He told me that when He died on the cross, everybody had sinned and everyone deserved to die, including me. But instead, He just wiped the slate clean, and if he hadn't done this for us, we would all perish in our sin.

Then I looked at my brother, and I saw a man in torment. I saw a man living with something that was killing him.

I said to him, " I forgive you."

The minute the words left my mouth, I began to feel great joy. I told him he needed to accept forgiveness from Jesus, so that he could move on with his life. He told me he did not think he could forgive himself. I said, " You're right, that's why you need God to do it for you."

After talking with my brother for about a half-hour I left to go home. Just as I was ready to drive off I heard the Lord speaking to me again. He said, "Now, accept the forgiveness I have for you." My eyes were opened. I could see that I was able not accept forgiveness because I was unwilling to forgive others. I needed forgiveness just as much as anyone else. I had always been able look at others and what they had done to me to justify my own anger, bitterness and unforgiveness. But now I knew I had to forgive in order to be forgiven and even that needed to come from power of the Lord and the work He did on the cross.

Truly it was finished. I was free.

The next morning my mother told me about the dream she had that night. She dreamed about an old lady standing in a church, clapping her hands and singing "The Holy Spirit is here." I took this as God's way of showing me that He had taken this dark affair, which could have destroyed my life, as well as someone very close to me, and He had turned it into one of the greatest discoveries of my life. Praise the Lord!

CHAPTER 36

I know there will be many challenges ahead to overcome. Especially now that I am a single parent. I hope that I can teach my children to make the right choices and learn to trust God. I hope we will all make it to heaven where we can live in peace with each other and leave the mess of this world behind.

As I journey through the rest of my life I wonder what God has in store for me and what other truths I will learn. I don't have to be afraid to go through the storms. I have discovered if I hang on tight to my Heavenly Father's hand, He will never let go of me.

I am continuing counseling. It has been invaluable to me. I've joined the Acoustic Neuroma Association, a support group for people who have had the same kind of tumor as I have. I am exercising and continuing with physical therapy on my own. After about a year, the left side of my face started to show some signs of movement. Still, I have accepted I will never look as I did before. I'm sure there will be other things I will have to let go of, but now I have the courage to look at myself and not let what's going on around me, or what other people are doing, to influence the choices that I make.

As I sit here at the end of telling my story I search for the words I want to say. I find myself only able to ask a question: What can a man say except, *"All things come from God."*

AUTHOR'S NOTE

Acoustic neuromas constitute 6 to 10% of all brain tumors. They are benign and are usually slow growing. They effect 1 in every 3,500 people. Twenty five years ago they were considered inoperable, however, today with surgery, there is only a 1% fatality rate. Scwann cells are what form an acoustic neuroma. They make up the lining of the eighth cranial nerve as it passes through a tiny canal which connects the inner ear to the brain. As they multiply they form a small mass which fills the canal. As the tumor expands, it extends into the brain, assuming a pear shape and putting pressure on tissue there. The symptoms can be hearing impairment in one ear, ear noise, and ear fullness. Other symptoms sometimes include unsteadiness, facial numbness or twitching. CT and MRI scans are used to make the final diagnosis. Depending on the extent of the tumor conditions of surgery almost always include one-sided hearing loss. Also, possibly tinnitus, facial weakness or paralysis, balance problems, eye discomfort and headaches. The size of my tumor and the length of my surgery was unusual.

Barbara Belknap has been president of the Portland, OR chapter of the Acoustic Neuroma Association for the past six years. She and the members this group have provided important support and frindship for me during my recovery. You may find out more about chapters in your area or information on acoustic neuromas by contacting: **Acoustic Neuroma Association, PO BOX 12402, Atlanta, GA 30355-2402, (404) 237-8023. E-mail: ana.usa.@aol.com. Web site: www.ana.usa.org**